D0232744

WHY
BREAST
FEEDING
MATTERS

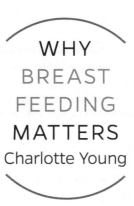

WHY
BREAST
FEEDING
MATTERS
Charlotte Young

pinter
&
martin

Why Breastfeeding Matters (Pinter & Martin Why It Matters 7)

First published by Pinter & Martin Ltd 2016

© 2016 Charlotte Young

Charlotte Young has asserted her moral right to be identified as the author of this work in accordance with the Copyright, Designs and Patents Act of 1988.

All rights reserved

ISBN 978-1-78066-520-7

Also available as ebook

Pinter & Martin Why It Matters ISSN ISSN 2056-8657

Series editor: Susan Last
Index: Helen Bilton
Design: Rebecca Longworth
Cover Design: Blok Graphic, London
Proofreader: Debbie Kennett

British Library Cataloguing-in-Publication Data
A catalogue record for this book is available from the British Library.

Set in Minion

Printed and bound in the UK by Ashford Colour Press Ltd, Gosport, Hampshire

This book has been printed on paper that is sourced and harvested from sustainable forests and is FSC accredited.

Pinter & Martin Ltd
6 Effra Parade
London SW2 1PS

pinterandmartin.com

Contents

Contents

To my parents, who are always there unconditionally and have made so much possible, even when at times my unconventional path through life must have confused the hell out of them. To those I love and live with, who have patiently endured hours of 'I'm writing'.

Thank you.

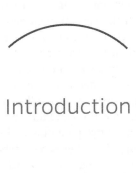

Introduction

This book isn't about extolling a list of all the 'benefits of breastfeeding', trying to convince people they should, or that they should feel bad if they don't. Nobody has the right to dictate to parents how they should raise their child, nor how a woman should use her body or for how long.

I believe in choice.

Choice is important because weeks, months or years down the line, the only people it really makes any difference to at all, the only ones left dealing with the emotions surrounding the experience of parenting a young baby – are the parents. It's *their* baby, *their* journey and *their* choices.

To make an informed choice parents need to know more than 'breast is best'. They need access to timely, accurate, evidence-based information (not just someone reaffirming what they believe to be true) and they also need effective, non-judgemental support when it matters. This is true whether their aim is to breastfeed for one feed or one year, and whether you agree with the choices they've made or not.

During pregnancy mums are often strongly encouraged to breastfeed, with the general message that it's optimal to breastfeed exclusively for six months to give their child the best possible start in life. This means that the baby is fed solely breastmilk, with no infant formula, water, other liquids or food. Parents aren't often told *why* this is recommended, beyond some vague spiel about the 'benefits'; perhaps baby will have fewer ear infections and tummy bugs, and it might help them score one or two points higher in terms of IQ…

When new mums find themselves, babe in arms, trying to establish breastfeeding, they quickly discover that breastfeeding 'support' is often a curious mixture of old wives' tales, myths and a touch of Harry Potter – every person they see offers a contradictory opinion. It's hard to believe at times that lactation is a well-studied biological function with its own academic journal.

Midwives trained decades ago are wheeled out as 'experts' in the media, even when their advice contradicts 30 years of sound science. Unless someone makes it clear that they are completely anti-breastfeeding, how can new parents decide who to believe, or tell good advice from bad?

Lactation barely gets a mention during the extensive training undertaken by paediatricians and other doctors, even from the perspective of the development of the immune system. This means there is a very real risk that breastfeeding may be perceived – by doctors and thus their patients – as not particularly significant or important, and that parents may be given inaccurate or ineffective information.

In our society most mothers do not breastfeed past the first few weeks, and many mothers don't know anyone who has breastfed without problems or for very long. Those who do establish breastfeeding and continue for several months or longer can feel self-conscious in public, and as if they need to cover up or go somewhere private. In this situation is it surprising that many mothers do not breastfeed their babies for as long as they initially intend? The odds are stacked against them.

What's more, breastfeeding is an emotive subject, because breasts are attached to a person. For some, their relationship with their body is so complex, or a previous experience so traumatic, that breastfeeding isn't an option. If a mum doesn't want to breastfeed, she doesn't need to explain or justify her decision to anyone. We have to respect her choice and help her explore acceptable alternatives – be that expressing milk, using donated milk or making formula feeding as safe as possible, in terms of its constituents, preparation and delivery.

Conversely, we must respect the rights and feelings of mothers who really want to breastfeed. Too many are told that it doesn't really matter, and that nowadays substitutes are nearly as good.

We have a healthcare system 'talking the talk' about breastfeeding, yet neither the system itself, nor society as a whole, is 'walking the walk'. Mothers are left picking up the pieces.

For those who really want to breastfeed, this all matters. I see it in grandmothers who become emotional recounting their own breastfeeding experiences – they are still carrying 'breastfeeding grief' and it mattered hugely to them. For many mothers the deep primal instinct to breastfeed their baby matters enormously, and the feelings they have about it affect them long after breastfeeding ends. In this book I aim to explain in more detail why this is.

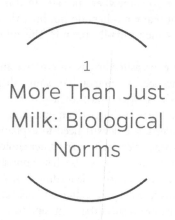

1
More Than Just Milk: Biological Norms

Many discussions of infant feeding are fundamentally flawed, because they're based on the assumption that breastfeeding is just about giving a baby the food they need to grow and develop. In this context, if the nutritional profile of different substances appears comparable, some may ask why or if breastfeeding actually matters at all. As a society we rarely talk about infant feeding beyond listing 'benefits' of breastfeeding, but there is so much more to it than that.

Sucking/suckling

Breastfeeding is the biological norm for human infants. While we often think of newborns as helpless, a healthy term baby born without the influence of drugs that can make them sleepy is equipped with a whole host of reflexes to enable them to feed. When placed on mum's chest, a newborn will gradually move towards the breast and locate the nipple using a combination of scent, sight, taste and touch, before self-attaching and feeding in an act often referred to as the 'breast crawl'. This is normal behaviour that is often prevented by interventions at birth.

These primitive reflexes, including sucking, originate in the central nervous system and gradually disappear or integrate as the baby matures. A young baby's suck reflex means he will instinctively suck anything that touches his lips or the roof of his mouth; helping to facilitate successful feeding. However, this reflex doesn't differentiate between the nipple or another trigger – as many parents who have found their baby sucking their collar, cheek or nose can testify. As a baby grows, sucking serves a number of purposes, from soothing to exploration of the environment, and it is a predominant activity during the first six months of life. The biologically normal way for these differing needs to be met is through continued breastfeeding. If we shift away from breastfeeding and instead use a bottle, which is not the biological norm, we need to recognise that there are knock-on effects. For example, a breastfeeding baby can choose to suckle but not transfer milk, but this isn't possible with a bottle. Thus, if we have a society where most people are mainly or exclusively formula feeding, we should expect that most people will use pacifiers (dummies) as well, to meet the normal suckling demands of a young baby; and this is seen in both the UK and the USA.

'Normal' is what we see every day around us, and what the majority of people do influences social acceptability. It takes no account of the biological norm. So if what parents see is that babies feed every three to four hours and use a pacifier (a nipple replica) in between, this is what they expect. When breastfed babies don't follow this predictable pattern, it can easily be perceived as a 'problem' that needs to be solved.

However, if we take breastfeeding as the biological norm, and examine pacifier use more closely, we see that moving away from the biological norm may have unintended consequences. Parents may not be aware that some studies have linked pacifiers with fewer breastfeeds and a shorter suckling duration per 24 hours (as we will learn later, this could impact on the amount of milk mum makes and baby's weight gain), shorter duration of exclusive breastfeeding and shorter total breastfeeding duration compared with no pacifier use, even in highly motivated mothers. While this effect isn't replicated in all studies, it may be a risk that a mum trying to establish feeding wants to factor into her decision-making process, particularly if the only reason mum wants to introduce a pacifier is because everyone does, rather than because she's desperately trying to soothe a fussy baby.

Mums may not always realise that they can choose to offer the breast to calm and soothe their baby at any time, instead of or as well as using a pacifier – even if formula is mainly or solely meeting baby's nutritional needs. This is rarely discussed, and many have never heard of it happening, so mums are often given no information about why they might want to even consider this approach.

Why might continuing to offer the breast as comfort, whether breastfeeding or formula-feeding, be worthwhile? The first and probably most obvious reason is that nipples don't need changing every few weeks and aren't regularly dropped on the floor at 2am, or accidentally left at home. They can soothe while waiting for a bottle to be ready or if baby won't accept a dummy.

Nipples also don't grow something called a biofilm – a slimy coating of bacteria that changes the normal bacterial balance of the mouth and is particularly resistant to antibiotics. In one study, researchers cultured 40 different species of bacteria from 10 used pacifiers; bacteria that are linked to a range of health conditions including candida (thrush), tooth decay and ear infections.

Pacifiers can also impact on oral development in terms of dentition. When a baby feeds at the breast, they don't suck the nipple. They should have a wide gape and a mouthful of breast so they can massage and milk the ducts. The breast adapts to the shape of the mouth, resulting in the nipple landing just before the spot on the roof of the mouth where the hard and soft palate meet. If you don't know where that is, feel around the roof of your own mouth with your tongue or thumb and note where it suddenly becomes soft.

Many are surprised at how far back this is, and it's easy to see that, in contrast, pacifiers and thumbs sit much further forward, resulting in a shift as to where pressure is applied. The late Dr Brian Palmer, a dentist specialising in the importance of breastfeeding for optimal oral development, showed that as the mouth has to adjust to any object inside it other than the breast, the unnatural forces generated by pacifier use can impact on the position of the teeth and the shape of the palate. This can encourage a habit of thrusting the tongue forward, and with excessive long-term use lead to speech problems and underdevelopment of the muscles in the jaw.

What all this means is that even if a baby is bottle-fed, or sometimes has a dummy, some breastfeeding can still help to increase the likelihood of normal oral development.

Security

The act of breastfeeding provides security for a newborn transitioning to life outside the womb. Encased in the sac of amniotic fluid, the baby is warm, cushioned and there's constant movement and muffled sound from mum's body and the outside world.

At birth, babies suddenly find themselves in an environment that is loud, bright and where much is completely unfamiliar – but not all. Held skin-to-skin, a baby can hear her mother's heartbeat and is comforted by familiar scents and tastes. Mum's chest secretes a substance that smells and tastes like amniotic fluid, providing a multi-sensory experience for her baby – like a Heston Blumenthal banquet.

There's a wonderful article by Dr Jenny Thomas MD, MPH, IBCLC, FAAP, FABM, entitled 'The Normal Newborn and Why Breastmilk is Not Just Food', that describes beautifully what newborns 'expect' as their biological norm. It's a must-read for any parent-to-be, as it describes why for babies, someone's chest is not only their preferred habitat, but also a logical choice in terms of where it makes sense to hang out. Mum's body increases blood flow to her chest area when baby is placed skin-to-skin, providing heat to keep him warm. There is also food and potential protection from predators (because tiny babies haven't yet realised that there are no wild animals lurking) and of course staying close reduces the odds of the baby getting lost or left behind, and increases their chances of easily accessing breastmilk when required.

Breastmilk further helps baby transition to life outside the womb by providing melatonin and nucleotides that help to regulate sleep and wake cycles.

Support during pain and illness

For both newborns and older babies, breastfeeding can prove invaluable when they are unwell. Breastmilk has high water content, and can usually continue when a baby is ill. A baby feeling under the weather may want to feed more frequently, while those who had previously reduced feeds may increase them again, or even return to exclusive breastfeeding for a few days.

This can help to reduce the risk of dehydration associated with sickness and diarrhoea or 'tummy bugs' (and the likelihood of needing hospitalisation), and exclusive breastmilk feeding is linked to a reduction in both severity and duration of this type of infection.

Breastfeeding and breastmilk are also recognised by the *British Medical Journal* as analgesics (pain relievers), and many mothers can testify as to its efficacy when babies receive vaccinations or are in pain from teething.

A 2006 article in the *International Breastfeeding Journal* explains how suckling and adsorption of fat from milk stimulates the release of a hormone that induces relaxation and pain relief during minor procedures.

> *The sweet flavour stimulates the release of opioids [which means it has an opiate-like effect, but isn't derived from opium] that decrease the perception of pain. Skin-to-skin contact stabilises baby's blood glucose levels, body temperature and respiration, reducing stress hormones and blood pressure. Lastly breastfeeding involves intimate social interaction which may result in a release of the anti-stress hormone oxytocin. These mechanisms of relaxation and pain relief work together.*

Some mums describe breastfeeding as being like a 'power hug', or a 'reset': a few short minutes on the breast seem to equate to much longer periods of other soothing activities such as rocking or cuddling. I've both experienced and witnessed grumpy babies who go to the breast for a couple of minutes and come off grinning.

More than just milk for mums too
Breastfeeding isn't just the biological norm for babies, it's also the physiological norm for mothers. Producing and providing milk for her baby is a primal, instinctive drive for some mums, and mothers who do not breastfeed need to know that there are physiological implications for them too.

From the moment of conception, a mother's breasts start to change in anticipation of feeding her baby. By the sixth month of pregnancy the system is complete; her body is primed and ready to go, both hormonally and physically.

When a mum finds herself in the position of not being able to breastfeed successfully, her feelings of sadness may be overwhelming and the experience may be traumatic.

One mum tried to express her feelings around breastfeeding:

> *My pregnancy was difficult and I didn't get the birth I wanted, so I was determined I was having breastfeeding. Even when it was all going wrong and things were terrible, I was more horrified by the thought of not breastfeeding. Looking back I was like someone with OCD, it wasn't at all rational and friends and family thought I was mad to carry on.*

Some mothers recall with disbelief how 'obsessive' they became about every drop of breastmilk, how emotionally invested they were in breastfeeding and how their journey really changed them as a person. Some start their next feeding relationship with a subsequent baby haunted by their previous experience. They tell me that mentally it was a dark time and that they can't risk going through that again. Some mothers use words like 'desperate', 'despair', 'heartbroken', 'devastated', 'traumatised', 'lost' and 'inconsolable' to describe how they felt while trying to fix their breastfeeding challenges.

We constantly hear that mums feel pressure to breastfeed, but to assume that external pressure is solely responsible for the emotions surrounding infant feeding totally underestimates the biological processes that are clearly at work.

Got milk?

When we talk about how many mums can or can't breastfeed,

we often look at quite a narrow picture; typically it's a group of mothers in a particular country or community, and we examine the percentage of mums capable of producing adequate amounts of milk when they feed their baby directly from the breast. However, the reality is much more complex than this.

Some mums can't feed at the breast because there's a medical concern, or the baby is premature; maybe the birth was traumatic and baby is simply refusing to latch, or mum can't find a way to achieve pain-free feeds. Some mums can or want to do some feeding but not all, and others may simply not want to put their baby to their breast, yet may still want to provide breastmilk.

Parents tell us that watching their baby grow and thrive on breastmilk can be extremely rewarding. Mums of premature babies (the most studied group) and younger mums report high satisfaction from providing milk, particularly when multiple other carers are involved in looking after the baby. Providing milk is something only they can do for their baby.

What all this tells us is that we should forget about trying to convince people to breastfeed, and instead focus on trying to effectively support those who want to do so. If more mums who initiated breastfeeding were helped to continue for as long as they wanted to, this in itself would provoke a shift in what we perceive as normal. Breastfeeding promotion isn't about trying to strong-arm people to breastfeed; it's about raising awareness of the fact that new mums aren't failing, they're being failed.

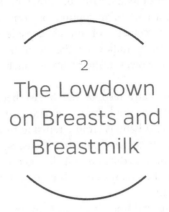

2
The Lowdown on Breasts and Breastmilk

At birth there is no difference between the male and female chest. If we think of a fully lactating breast as a tree in bloom, all babies are born with the seed planted but dormant. In many females the beginning of a breast bud is the first physical sign of puberty. As hormones like oestrogen and progesterone are released, the seed is given the right conditions to grow.

Over the coming years, glands (which is where milk may later be made) and ducts (hollow stalk-like pipes that transport milk from the glands to the openings on the end of the nipple) are laid down – these structures are the mechanics of lactation. The hormonal peaks of each menstrual cycle provoke continued growth, until the seed has become the 'primary ductal tree'. In gardening terms the breast is now most comparable to a new tree in spring: it has branches and buds, but hasn't yet developed leaves or flowers.

The most rapid, noticeable growth of the breasts typically occurs within the first four years after the onset of puberty, when hormones are most abundant. After this many women report further changes even years later, particularly with weight fluctuations. This is because the spaces around the ducts and glands are filled with fatty and connective tissues. The size of a non-lactating breast is largely determined by the amount of fat it contains.

Pregnancy triggers the final stage of development to enable lactation (milk production). Hormone levels shift significantly, triggering further development of the glands and ducts, alongside a reduction in the surrounding fatty tissues. Some mums don't feel obvious changes until the last trimester or after birth, while others notice significant differences just weeks into pregnancy – both are normal. Increased blood flow to breasts and nipples may be obvious, as blue veins develop close to the surface of the skin and areolas darken. This is thought to provide the baby with a clear visual target.

By around the eighth month of pregnancy, the profile of bacteria living on the skin around mum's nipples changes, and a specific species of 'good bacteria' called *Bifidobacterium* can be found. Initially scientists were confused by this discovery, as this particular bacterium is anaerobic and can't survive when exposed to air. What they discovered was that the bacteria thrive deep inside the oxygen-free environment of the milk ducts, before being secreted via invisible droplets of colostrum (see below). Although the bacteria can't survive, they leave behind potent acids and antibiotic chemicals that could repel potentially dangerous organisms such as *Staphylococcus aureus*.

So by the time the baby is born, the breast is comparable to a tree in summer. The structures involved in lactation now fill the breast, and as soon as hormone levels shift again with delivery of the placenta, full milk production can commence.

Colostrum

- The 'milk' produced from around the middle of pregnancy and immediately after giving birth is called colostrum. While some mums leak drops during pregnancy, others don't have any outward indication it's there until after giving birth.
- This thick, yellowy/orange substance is highly concentrated and so a baby only needs small amounts of approximately 2–10ml or ½–2 teaspoons per feed, totalling around 30ml (6 tsp or 1 ounce) in the first 24 hours after birth.
- Colostrum is considered extremely important for the newborn immune system as it provides white blood cells called macrophages (or 'big eaters'). These cells are known to help destroy a whole range of potentially dangerous bacteria. It's also rich in antibodies, which coat the lining of baby's immature intestines and act as a barrier against harmful pathogens.
- This is why many refer to colostrum as 'baby's first vaccine', and even if they're not planning to breastfeed longer term some mums decide to feed it to the baby (either by breastfeeding, or expressing and feeding it to the baby with a syringe or teaspoon) before switching to formula feeding.
- Hand-expressing small amounts and freezing them ready for birth can be helpful if your healthcare provider feels there's an increased likelihood baby may need feeding with more urgency than usual after birth (for example, if mum has gestational diabetes).

Transitional milk

- Between two and five days after birth, colostrum becomes 'transitional milk'. This is often referred to (rather inaccurately) as milk 'coming in'. Volumes become more copious due to increasing water content and fat levels and overall calorie content increases too. Visually it looks like a creamy/orange liquid and the colour can vary widely from pale to resembling orange juice.

- This ties in with a typical term baby's increasing needs, which are estimated at 1–3 tsp on day two, increasing gradually to 30–60ml (1–2oz) per feed by the end of day three.

- Some mums notice a sudden increase in milk production and wake up with full, firm, heavy breasts, often referred to as 'physiological engorgement'. It's normal for them to feel warm and it can take a week or so to settle.

- If mum feels unwell or has breasts that are extremely hot, red, shiny or so hard baby can't latch easily, it's worth asking a midwife or breastfeeding support worker for help. This type of engorgement is called 'pathological' and helpers can check that the baby is well attached, removing enough milk and feeding frequently enough. Sometimes this type of engorgement occurs as a result of over-hydration in mum due to IV fluids (given via drip) during labour and delivery. In this instance mum will often carry excess water in other parts of her body too, so her feet, ankles and hands may appear swollen and feel uncomfortable.

- Other mums experience a more gradual increase to full supply over several days. If baby is feeding well they may not experience the excessive leaking described by others; both are normal.

- Full milk production is triggered by delivery of the

placenta and happens whether or not a mum plans to breastfeed. Midwives can advise on the most effective ways to suppress milk if mum doesn't wish to continue lactating, and explain what's normal versus what might indicate a problem, such as an infection that might require treatment.

- Transitional milk is packed with antibodies that fight infection and support the development of the baby's immune system.

- Once milk volumes have increased, maintaining supply becomes about milk removal: the more milk the baby takes and the more frequently they feed, the more milk is produced. If mum's breasts are very full and milk is not removed, production slows down and will eventually cease.

- If mum is exclusively expressing, using a double hospital-grade pump followed by a few minutes of hand-expressing has been shown to be very effective in removing more milk, which can help to maintain or increase supply. The Stanford School of Medicine has produced some excellent expressing video tutorials, details of which can be found at the end of the book. Some mums, however, just don't get along with a pump, and find hand-expressing more effective and less time-consuming; there really are no hard and fast rules.

Mature milk

- By around the end of the second week, milk is considered mature. It is typically thinner and more watery-looking than transitional milk; this doesn't indicate that the milk isn't rich or fatty enough.

- Breastmilk can also have a blue hue, which again

is normal: human milk proteins look different to those in cow's milk that we are used to seeing. What's more, it can sometimes look a different colour if mum is taking medication; some herbal supplements can turn milk greenish, while foods like beetroot can give it a purple tinge!

- Mature milk continues to contain protective antibodies, as well as an array of other constituents that we will discuss in more detail later.

- Engorgement and excessive fullness should typically settle, although it's normal for some mums to still leak milk between feeds (others never do, and that's also normal). This often settles at around six weeks, when some mums can suddenly feel less full and worry that their supply has dropped. All mums are different and some continue to need breast pads for much longer.

The mechanics of the breast

I meet a lot of mums who don't fully understand how milk production works. They may have heard that they need to let their breasts 'refill' between feeds, or they may worry that their supply has dwindled if they don't feel overly full.

Some people like to compare breastfeeding to a factory rather than a warehouse, as milk production is always ongoing. This is partly true, but it's probably more accurate to say that it's like an efficient factory with a warehouse attached.

When the 'factory' of thousands of tiny glands (called alveoli) in mum's breast produces milk, it's stored in clusters of tiny sacs that resemble bunches of grapes. When the milk ejection reflex or 'letdown' is triggered, muscles contract to push milk out of these cells and down the tubes or ducts that lead to the nipple opening. Milk may also move into the ducts and can start dripping or leaking from the nipple.

If adequate milk isn't removed from the warehouse, it starts backing up. Breasts start to feel firmer as pressure in the ducts increases, and noticeable and uncomfortable lumps or hard sections of the breast start to form in areas that become overly full.

We now have, in effect, a traffic jam in the breast, which can halt the flow of blood and lymph (a clear fluid that circulates through tissues to cleanse them, before draining away through the lymphatic system). As a result tissues become over-saturated, resulting in swelling (oedema) and engorgement, or 'non-infectious mastitis'.

If some milk is removed, but not enough to clear the traffic jam, or some areas are left without enough milk removed, mum may find some areas of her breast feel softer while other sections remain lumpy and tender. If one particular duct has been under strain and has become clogged with milk that hasn't released, this is often referred to as a blocked or plugged duct.

Milk that does not move through the breast appropriately results in milk stasis, or 'milk sitting about'. This, combined with the reduced flow of lymph, can increase the risk of developing an infection, known as 'infectious mastitis'.

The key with any over-fullness or blockage is to remove milk as quickly and as efficiently as possible. Applying gentle pressure to hard or blocked areas when feeding or expressing can often help release some or all of the milk, but if breasts regularly don't feel soft, floppy and relieved of their 'warehouse stash' after feeding, seek support to find out why.

In terms of maintaining a good milk supply, adequate milk removal is important because when the breasts become very full, a protein and a hormone in the milk communicate with the factory to slow down and eventually cease production.

Breastmilk facts
- Breastmilk is not a dairy product, because mum is not a cow. Having a dairy allergy or intolerance in the family doesn't mean you can't breastfeed. We know that when mums consume dairy, the proteins can sometimes be found in breastmilk – therefore, if necessary, avoiding dairy makes breastmilk free from dairy protein too.
- Breastmilk is a live substance like blood. It's made up of thousands of constituents that change from minute to minute, hour to hour and week to week.
- Acute changes occur in lactose, glucose, sodium, potassium, and chloride levels 5–6 days before and 6–7 days after maternal ovulation; it is not yet known why.

The message is 'what's already here isn't being used, so don't make much more'.

When milk is effectively and frequently removed (reducing the stash in the warehouse), the body sends signals telling the factory that the production rate can increase again. As the production plant becomes established, the staff become more efficient at predicting demand and the warehouse is less likely to be overwhelmed with excess milk.

When the breast is drained of its initial store, the factory can continue to supply milk as it is produced, at a drip, drip rate – so the warehouse is never truly 'empty'. Storage capacity can be thought of as warehouse size (although this doesn't correlate with breast size). The factory is still capable of producing the same amount of milk, but mums with a smaller warehouse may need to 'ship out' milk more frequently, both for their own comfort and to meet baby's needs. This is just one reason why scheduled breastfeeds will appear to work for some mothers and not others.

While we're on the subject of milk-producing capability, it's interesting to note that a study in the 1980s found that well-nourished Australian mothers feeding twins could produce 2,100ml (approximately 74oz) of breastmilk per 24 hours. Some mums successfully breastfeed triplets, so if we consider that a single baby needs a maximum of around 900ml (around 32oz) in 24 hours, most mums aren't running anywhere near the limits of what they're capable of producing.

What's normal and why does it hurt?

When babies are effectively breastfeeding they don't suck, they suckle. This is an action during which baby tips their head back, opens their mouth wide (like a yawn), brings their tongue forward over the gum ridge and attaches deeply: not to the nipple, but to the breast. The nipple lands far back in the mouth, just before the junction with the soft palate, where the roof of your mouth becomes soft.

Baby needs to be held in a position that comfortably enables her to continue to do all of the above, without straining or turning to reach for the duration of the feed. Her chin needs to snuggle deep into the breast, with her head well tipped back to leave her nose clear.

In order to transfer milk effectively (and for mum's comfort), baby needs to stay in this position – with her mouth open wide and tongue forward – for the whole feed, to continue to transfer milk after the first couple of minutes. After baby triggers the milk ejection reflex or 'letdown', she then needs to undulate her tongue in an action that resembles a wave, called 'peristalsis'.

As the back of the tongue drops, the seal she has created with the deep attachment results in a negative pressure that pulls milk from the breast. She then raises the back of the tongue to shift the milk into her throat for swallowing, before dropping it again to pull more milk and so on. This should result in a 'suck, pause (mouth filling), swallow' sequence. Babies who are a bit less organised or effective may end up coughing, spluttering or clicking as they struggle to regulate the flow. This can cause problems with fitting breathing into the sequence, which can leave them panting like they've been running. Some might bunch up the back of their tongue, or pull back to a more shallow latch to try to deal with milk that is now landing at the front of their mouth instead of the back.

Although there can be many reasons for pain while breastfeeding, or baby never appearing satisfied, the most common issues are:

- Baby is not attaching deeply to the breast. This can result in the nipple ending up much further forward in his mouth where it can be quashed against the hard palate. This can cause pain, trauma and reduce the milk flow to baby much like squishing a straw would. He may not be tipping his head back well, opening his mouth wide or keeping his tongue forward, resulting in a shallower latch and a disorganised or uncoordinated sucking and swallowing pattern. He may not be doing the correct action with his tongue because of something like a tongue tie (where the piece of skin underneath the tongue is too short or too far forward – this can be quickly and easily resolved in babies), or because of a difficult delivery.
- Thrush (candida) – a fungal infection of the nipple. The risk of this increases if mum was particularly prone to infections like vaginal thrush pre-pregnancy, or if she takes antibiotics (including during a caesarean section). Thrush is typically treated with an

appropriate anti-fungal medication.

- Blockages behind the nipple/areola area. Small blocked ducts can cause a burning sensation when feeding for some mothers.
- Mastitis. Pain in the breasts can be caused by a breast infection; either from insufficient milk being removed or perhaps from damage to the nipple which has provided an entry point for infection. Mum will typically have a high temperature, feel fluish and unwell. It's important to seek medical support; antibiotics may be needed in some cases to prevent an abscess developing.

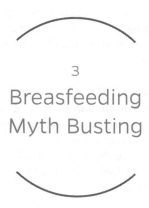

3

Breasfeeding Myth Busting

There are many myths surrounding breastfeeding that refuse to die, despite research consistently demonstrating that they are untrue.

Myth 1: You have no way of knowing how much baby is actually drinking

Many parents worry that it's impossible to know how much a breastfed baby is drinking, and some turn to formula because they want to be able to 'see' how much the baby is getting. However, there are a number of ways to tell how much milk a breastfed baby is getting. Firstly, we can establish how to recognise 'active drinking', when the baby receives lots of milk quickly and easily, compared to 'nibbling', a much faster, shallower sucking pattern that results in baby receiving much smaller amounts in return for the energy he expends. Parents who can tell when their babies are consistently swallowing large mouthfuls of milk are much less worried about the exact amount that's going in.

Next we can look at output, because what goes in must come out. Looking at a baby's nappies will give us an indication of whether she is drinking enough milk in the early days. Here is what should happen:

Day 1 (first 24 hours of life)
Pees: At least once or more in the first 24 hours. Newborns may have urine that is orange- or pink-tinged due to urate crystals, and this is normal at this stage.

Poos: At least once in the first 24 hours. At this stage it is called meconium. It looks like tar and is very dark green/brown/black and sticky.

Day 2
Pees: At least twice.

Poos: At least one large or two smaller. Typically still meconium, becoming less sticky, thinner and turning greener.

Day 3-4
Pees: Three times or more; the amount of wee increases and the nappies feel heavier than before.

Poos: Three or more. These now become 'transitional stools' and are lighter and thinner, toffee-coloured brown.

Day 5 onwards
Pees: Five or more heavy nappies per day.

Poos: At least two large or three to four smaller soft stools (the size of a £2 coin) or more per day.

Breastfed baby poo is mustard-yellow in colour and may contain little pieces that look like seeds or cottage cheese. It will be looser than the more formed poo of an older child, but shouldn't be excessively runny or thin.

The only problem with using output as an indicator is the element of subjectivity. How wet is wet? How big does the poo need to be? Nonetheless, it's still important. A baby not pooing or transitioning through the above steps as expected should be assessed to see if they are feeding effectively.

Is your newborn getting enough milk?

- As nappies can be very absorbent and newborns only pee small amounts, it's not always easy in the early days to tell if a nappy is wet. Placing a piece of soft toilet paper inside a clean nappy can make it easier to tell.
- Pour three tablespoons of water (45ml) into a dry nappy; this is roughly how much urine your baby should pass after the first 5–6 days.
- As a general rule of thumb, in the first five days expect the same number of wet and dirty nappies as the baby is days old. Baby may have 2–3 very large stools to replace 4–5 smaller ones, while others go after each feed and that's fine too.

Call your healthcare provider if:

- Baby is having fewer wet or dirty nappies than outlined above.
- Baby has dark-coloured poo after day four. By this point poo should be mustard-yellow or well on the way.
- Baby has dark-coloured urine after day 3 (should be pale yellow to clear).
- Baby is sleepy and difficult to rouse to feed.
- You have any other concerns about your baby's intake.

The next indicator of milk intake is what is happening overall and whether baby is fussy or unsettled, particularly around day 2. If baby isn't transferring enough milk at this point, the vast majority of term, healthy babies will try to let you know. They tend to cry a lot. They repeatedly don't settle after feeding, or take a really short feed before falling asleep quickly, but rouse and signal again as soon as they're moved slightly. Some stay at the breast hour after hour and parents often feel things aren't going exactly as they should.

Healthy, term babies, without jaundice, don't typically fall asleep at the breast in the middle of swallowing large amounts of milk. Babies most often fall asleep when they're not 'actively drinking' – either because they've had a good hit of milk, or because the amount they're able to transfer has become too small to be worth staying awake burning energy for. Parents are often told to tickle their baby, blow on them or undress them, but gently squeezing or 'compressing' the breast, pushing colostrum or milk down to the baby, can often have their eyes popping back open as they realise the milk is still flowing.

It's normal for newborns to sometimes fall asleep before they've taken a full feed, perhaps after a good period of drinking as they've become warm and relaxed. A quick nappy change can often rouse them again to continue and finish the feed.

Not drinking quite enough milk is problematic for small babies, as this alone can make them disorganised and less effective when they do feed, exacerbating the problem. For some babies taking less than they need can quickly make it harder for them to latch well and stay awake. It may be that all that's needed is something as simple as a tweak to positioning, or it could be, if baby is persistently only managing a shallower latch and 'nibbling' for some reason, that in the short-term they need some extra colostrum or milk supplemented back to help.

If a baby isn't getting enough milk, his mouth and lips

gradually become dry and, if you offer a finger to suck, the inside of his mouth may feel dry too. His fontanelle may appear sunken and his cry may sound hoarse; some liken the sound to that made by a pterodactyl. This means baby needs some additional milk supplemented straight away – be that breastmilk, expressed breastmilk, donated milk or formula, and urgent breastfeeding support is needed.

If a baby doesn't receive fluids at this point, he will eventually run out of energy to signal his hunger and start to sleep for longer periods. Depending on the degree of weight loss some babies can be supplemented with milk, while others may need slower rehydration. Seeking medical assistance is vital.

Myth 2: Breastfeeding can cause saggy breasts

We repeatedly hear that breastfeeding causes breasts to sag – despite the fact that numerous studies have confirmed this isn't the case. Drooping breasts are actually linked to:

- Age. As people get older, gravity takes its toll.
- Higher BMI and large pre-pregnancy breasts.
- Greater number of pregnancies.
- Smoking
- Genetics

A 2012 study examining the breasts of twins found that moisturising, hormone replacement therapy and breastfeeding *improved* skin quality and appearance.

Whether you breastfeed or not, the same physical and hormonal changes take place during pregnancy as the breasts prepare to produce milk. When baby is born, engorgement or fullness typically peaks when milk 'comes in', and can cause stretching of the skin in the same way that the abdominal skin in pregnancy stretches as baby grows.

For those with implants, a 2013 study by a plastic surgeon

found breastfeeding didn't affect the look of surgically enlarged breasts, concluding:

> *Women are free to breastfeed without the concern of affecting the appearance of their breast augmentation. Since nursing is beneficial for a mother's and child's overall health, it's important to convey this message to new mothers.*

The 'saggy boob' myth may stem from the fact that when breastfeeding is reduced and eventually ceases (whether after a few weeks, or a few years), breasts undergo a process called 'involution'.

Whereas during pregnancy ducts and milk-producing glands swell and grow, during involution they shrink and the proportion of fat and connective tissue increases again. It is estimated to take between six months and three years for this transition to be complete, so what your breasts look like weeks or even months after stopping feeding may not be indicative of the end result.

Breasts that have just stopped lactating are often soft, floppy and droopy or, to quote one mum, 'like a spaniel's ears'. At this point the process of 'rebuilding' the non-lactating breast has only just started.

Myth 3: Many mums can't make enough milk
One of the most common reasons mums give for stopping breastfeeding is that they (or those around them) think that they are not producing enough milk for the baby. These mums can be split into a few different groups:

- Perceived problem: mum is making and baby is drinking normal amounts of milk, but due to different expectations mum may believe there's a problem. It could be that mum expects to feed every 4 hours, but baby wants to feed every 2-3. It could be baby is having a normal fussy spell and feeding lots, but the parents haven't been told to expect this.

- Babies increase milk supply by feeding more frequently than normal, and common times for doing this are at around 3, 5, 12 and 16 weeks. These periods are often called 'growth spurts', although some consider it a misleading term as physical growth doesn't always occur. As a result some prefer the term 'fussy spell'. Even bottlefed babies can have these spells and fuss more when feeding, suddenly taking to feeding little and often for a couple of days. It's thought to be a combination of a developmental spurt and the need to prompt an increase in milk supply for the weeks ahead.

- Sometimes baby can be unsettled and want to feed frequently, as though ravenous, even when weight gain and feeding have been great. This generally lasts a few days before passing, but it's not uncommon for mums to believe they have simply run out of milk or are not producing enough.

- Transfer issue without a supply problem: these mums experience a normal start to lactation, with typical volumes of milk 'coming in', but baby simply can't transfer enough.

- Transfer issue with a supply problem: these mums experience a normal start to lactation with typical volumes of milk 'coming in', but because the baby can't transfer enough, her supply has dropped.

- Reduced supply: these mums don't experience an increase to full milk production during the normal period, but do produce some milk. This might be due to a problem that can be resolved, such as small fragments of placenta retained after delivery, thyroid issues or unstable blood sugars following gestational diabetes. Or it may be due to a hormonal condition, or because mum has insufficient glandular tissue.

- Delayed, absent or failed lactation: milk volumes have not increased at all post-partum, or mum is unable to produce any breastmilk. Again this can be caused by something that can be treated, like retained placenta or hormonal imbalance, but at other times no obvious reason can be found. Unfortunately, there is very little research done, as we seem happy to accept that 'some mothers just aren't made to make milk'.

Most problems fall into the first three categories, which can often be addressed and resolved.

When it comes to slow weight gain in babies, the baby not being able to feed well enough is much more common than insufficient breastmilk production. However, some of these babies are 'feeding', or should I say 'hanging out at the breast', for inordinate amounts of time. Everyone wrongly believes they are eating well, and if they don't gain weight it must be because there isn't enough milk.

There's an analogy here with fertility. Most mums conceive naturally within a year; however, we also recognise that it takes some couples longer, and that some mums don't conceive naturally. We don't judge people on their fertility or their ability to procreate, and we know support and fertility treatment to conceive may be required. We also acknowledge that in some cases treatment isn't successful, and they may not be able to conceive at all.

Milk production is in some ways comparable. Most mums can easily produce the amount of milk baby needs; however, some may feel they have to work hard to increase or maintain a full supply. Similarly, some mums don't produce enough breastmilk naturally; support and treatment to help them produce more or enough milk may be required. We also have to recognise that there is still a percentage of people for whom support won't work, and that some mothers simply can't lactate.

Myth 4: Breastfeeding always hurts at the start until nipples have 'toughened up'

No, no, no! Toughen up? Do women need to have leather nipples to lactate successfully? This pervasive myth means it's not uncommon for women to tell me they had the 'normal pain and cracked nipples you expect at the beginning'.

Yes, breasts may be sensitive or tender for a few seconds at the start of a feed – particularly in the very early days as baby develops coordination and because it's a new sensation – but it shouldn't be toe-curling agony or cause any sort of damage to the nipple.

If the baby has the breast in the right place in his mouth and is doing the right action there is nothing to cause pain and damage. However, if his latch is shallow he could pinch or squash the sensitive nipple tissue, which can cause the nipple to turn white or blue temporarily after a feed (vasospasm). Some mums get a stripe or ridge top to bottom, while others find that post-feed their nipple looks squashed like a new lipstick. Some say they can feel their baby 'biting' or 'chewing', or note an irritating rubbing. This can disturb blood flow and result in stabbing pains after a feed, often mistaken for thrush. Friction can cause soreness and the areola may become red, itchy and flaky; these are also symptoms of fungal infections.

Whoever is providing breastfeeding support needs to be skilled enough to establish why there's a problem and to find the best way to help resolve things. Several studies have confirmed the importance of correcting early sucking problems, and working out whether feeding pain is going to self-resolve over a few days or weeks, or whether there is something more going on.

Often mothers are told to 'stick at it', even when it should have been clear from early on that things were not going to magically and spontaneously improve. Or they are given endless suggestions of things to try, without anyone really understanding what the problem is.

Some mums I see comment that they had damage in the early days, but it healed and didn't reoccur. Some say they had pain, but after a number of weeks it eased or became bearable; they may still have problems, which is why they're seeing me, but now maybe weight gain is slow, or baby never appears settled or suffers from reflux.

Some believe that once nipples have healed it means the baby is therefore feeding 'optimally', which may fuel the myth that nipples' toughen up'. If the primary function of breasts is to lactate, it makes little biological sense for the majority of women to have to endure unbearable pain to perform this function.

Myth 5: If you're breastfeeding you should eat a perfect diet
What is a 'perfect diet' anyway? No coffee or alcohol, no strong flavours like garlic, or greens, or citrus or chocolate… if we believed every food myth there would be nothing left for breastfeeding mums to eat! Contrary to popular belief, breastmilk isn't made from the contents of mum's stomach, but from her blood. While it's advisable to eat a typical balanced diet, as in pregnancy, this is true however a mum feeds her baby. Vitamin and mineral levels in breastmilk are remarkably consistent between women, regardless of their diets. A mother's body will take what it needs to produce breastmilk from her stores, pulling calcium from bones and fat from reserves. We know that in countries where food is

scarce and diets are limited, mums still produce good-quality breastmilk. Let's tackle a few of the things breastfeeding mothers are warned to avoid:

Alcohol

The amount of alcohol that passes into breastmilk is a microscopic fraction of that consumed by the mother. The level of alcohol peaks in blood and breastmilk approximately ½–1 hour after drinking and does not accumulate over time. Alcohol leaves breastmilk as it leaves the blood. Dr Jack Newman, a Canadian paediatrician and breastfeeding specialist, writes:

> *Reasonable alcohol intake should not be discouraged at all. As is the case with most drugs, very little alcohol comes out in the milk. The mother can take some alcohol and continue breastfeeding as she normally does. Prohibiting alcohol is another way we make life unnecessarily restrictive for nursing mothers.*

Carlos González, a Spanish paediatrician and breastfeeding specialist, agrees:

> *The legal driving limit in the UK is 0.08 per cent. If your alcohol level is higher than 0.15 per cent you are unmistakably drunk. If it goes above 0.55 per cent you simply drop dead. Therefore, it's absolutely impossible for breastmilk to contain more than 0.55 per cent alcohol. Alcohol-free beer can legally contain nearly double this level – up to 1 per cent alcohol. Consequently, even the breastmilk of a completely inebriated mother could be bottled and labelled 'alcohol free'.*

Both authors stress that heavy regular drinking and breastfeeding isn't advisable, but heavy drinking and *parenting* isn't advisable. A breastfeeding mother having a few drinks is unlikely to be a problem, but if you're planning on getting rip-roaring drunk it's probably not safe to be holding or caring for a baby, whether you breastfeed or bottle-feed.

Caffeine

Most breastfeeding mums can drink moderate amounts of caffeine. Studies suggest that a dose of caffeine comparable to a cup of coffee results in breastmilk containing around 1 per cent of mum's level, and peaks around an hour after consumption.

Many people are not aware that caffeine therapy is used in premature babies, to aid lung development and reduce the incidence of episodes of apnoea (where baby temporarily stops breathing due to an immature central nervous system), as well as to help wean babies from mechanical ventilation.

One study examining breastmilk after maternal caffeine consumption concluded that the amount of caffeine ingested via breastmilk was small compared to the therapeutic dose babies could be given directly.

Another study examined consumption of 500mg of caffeine per day (equivalent to around five 8oz cups of standard coffee), compared to mums who drank decaffeinated:

> *Serum did not contain detectable amounts of caffeine on the last day of either experimental period. Performance during the caffeine and no-caffeine periods was not significantly different with respect to either 24-hour heart rate or sleep time.*

What's also interesting is a small experiment that showed large variability in caffeine metabolism. Babies younger than a few months don't metabolise caffeine as well as adults, and a range of between 8 to 41 hours was identified. Another study found that during pregnancy, babies exposed to caffeine only responded with more activity and wakefulness if mum didn't regularly consume it; an effect which may continue after birth. Some babies do appear to be more sensitive to caffeine in mum's diet when breastfeeding, perhaps if mum drinks more than average and baby is a slow metaboliser. If a baby is jittery, irritable, wide-eyed or fussy it might be worth eliminating caffeine for a week to see if baby is reacting. Most mums who drink normal amounts of coffee will see no effects in their babies.

Dairy

Dairy intolerance, or cow's milk protein intolerance (CMPI), is a hot topic in the breastfeeding world, partly because the condition is used in marketing by the formula companies, which promote expensive hypoallergenic formulas that can also be prescribed by doctors and paediatricians. A tin of hypoallergenic formula such as Neocate costs around £30 and lasts approximately 2½ days; the cost of hypoallergenic formula to the NHS is around £5,000 per year for each baby who gets it. Of course there are some babies that suffer from dairy allergy or intolerance, and it goes without saying that it's crucial they have access to suitable milk, be that prescribed formula or breastmilk when mum is supported to eliminate foods from her diet. Some babies turn out to be intolerant to other ingredients in some formulas; recipes differ and for some switching to another brand will resolve problems. In clinic I have suggested numerous babies be seen by a health professional to discuss the possibility of intolerance to their current formula – but it's a huge leap from there to the current position, where every mention of a crying baby results in people suggesting it's probably dairy in mum's diet that's the issue.

One mum said:

> *After a feeding assessment I was told to cut dairy, chocolate and several other items out of my diet ASAP and contact the doctor for reflux medication. Several days later I discovered my baby was gulping air at the breast. As soon as we stopped this, the projectile vomit also immediately stopped! I didn't modify my diet but felt I was being blamed for my baby's reflux because of what I was eating.*

This is problematic because:

- For some mums cutting dairy from their diet seems so difficult that they're more likely to switch to a hypoallergenic formula, believing their milk is responsible for baby's problems. If fussiness was caused by breastfeeding technique rather than CMPI, using a bottle with hypoallergenic formula may resolve the issue even if dairy wasn't the key piece of the puzzle. These babies are thus at an unnecessary nutritional disadvantage.
- Cutting dairy can reduce in a drastic calorie drop for mums. Dairy can contribute significantly to energy intake and many busy mums who cut dairy aren't told they need to replace the calories by eating nuts, healthy fats and other nutritious foods. A sudden, severe calorie drop can result in a milk supply drop.
- Removing dairy may mask another problem. Here's my theory based on experience (anecdote): we know dairy proteins are harder to digest than human milk proteins. If baby has a digestive issue –perhaps they're swallowing air from a shallow latch on the breast or bottle teat, are crying excessively and have wind or colic – digesting more complex proteins on top may become problematic. If we remove the protein, we may

make digestion easier and thus see an improvement in gut-related symptoms. As the baby starts feeding effectively, they become more capable of digesting cow's milk proteins without problem.

We also need to ask, does the baby really have reflux? An interesting paper entitled 'Excessive crying and gastro-oesophageal reflux disease in infants: misalignment of biology and culture', says:

Excessive crying is the most common problem presenting to the doctor in the first months of life in western industrialised societies, affecting up to 30% of infants. There has been an exponential increase in the diagnosis of gastro-oesophageal reflux disease (GORD) in babies who cry excessively over the past few decades, and many parents believe their crying infant 'has reflux'.

The authors go on to say that infant-care practices in western industrialised societies have shifted towards an emphasis on infant autonomy, yet biologically the baby is an 'exterogestate foetus' (an immature infant that continues to be nurtured outside the womb) for at least the first six months of life. Newborns are dependent on maternal co-regulation (close contact with their mothers that helps develop their biological capabilities) for optimal function – a period often referred to as 'the fourth trimester'. The paper hypothesises that in many cases 'reflux' is a physiological manifestation of a misalignment between biology and culture. The authors propose that infants who cry excessively may be predisposed to reflux after three to four months of age:

If this hypothesis is correct, an integrated clinical approach to crying babies less than three to four months of age that considers feeding management (e.g., frequent feeds, breast- or bottle-feeding technique, referral to a lactation consultant, cow's milk allergy), parental responsiveness (e.g., prompt response to infant cues), sensory nourishment (e.g., sling or backpack, walks, massage) and sleep management (e.g., nocturnal co-sleeping) should, firstly, decrease crying when applied to infants less than three to four months of age, and secondly, decrease the incidence of GORD in these infants once they are older than three to four months of age.

The UK's NICE guidance on the treatment of reflux agrees:

In breast-fed infants with frequent regurgitation associated with marked distress, ensure that a person with appropriate expertise and training carries out a breastfeeding assessment.

Some babies are intolerant and need dairy removing from their diet. However, for most a full feeding assessment is a more appropriate first-line treatment than drastic dietary changes for the mother or medication for the baby.

Strong flavours and gas or wind-causing foods (garlic, spices, herbs, cabbage, broccoli and beans)
Many people believe that foods that can cause flatulence in mum can cause her breastfed baby to suffer from wind. However, intestinal gas is produced when gut bacteria meet intestinal fibre, and neither of these can pass into breastmilk. Others believe that mums need a 'bland diet' to make breastmilk 'more digestible'; this is simply an old wives' tale. In fact babies

enjoy different tastes and flavours and experience these in the womb via amniotic fluid and while breastfeeding. It's one of the disadvantages of formula that the taste is the same at every single feed.

Several studies have shown that different foods can flavour breastmilk. Danish scientists found that liquorice flavour peaked strongly in breastmilk two hours after mum ingested a capsule, as did caraway seed flavour. Mint appeared at lower concentrations but peaked much later, at six hours after ingestion; banana flavour didn't come through in breastmilk at all. The authors of the study theorised that flavour exposure could prepare babies for the wide range of foods they are likely to encounter once they are weaned:

> *During infancy and childhood, individuals are very receptive to sensory and cognitive learning, and the behaviors established in this period are most probably important for later preference and food behaviors.*

In a second series of experiments the same authors explored whether breastfed babies were more likely to eat certain meals than babies fed on formula from a bottle. Researchers exposed babies to caraway via breastmilk, then gave both formula and breastfed babies meals laced with caraway flavouring. The results were interesting. The breastfed babies were happier eating meals containing caraway flavouring than babies fed on formula. Feeding caraway purée to breastfed babies didn't further increase acceptance rate, but feeding it to the formula fed babies did. The lead author concluded:

> *Diet does change the flavouring of the milk, but it's not like if the mother eats apple pie, the infant thinks, 'Mmm, apple pie', and gets to like it. It seems that*

*breastfed infants get used to small flavour changes and
so they become more accepting of a variety of flavours
compared to formula-fed infants.*

What's more, it seems that babies may enjoy these varying
flavours. A study in the 1990s found that, when mothers
maintained a bland diet and then took a garlic supplement,
their infants spent on average 30.8 per cent longer feeding.
The more regularly garlic was eaten, the less pronounced
the effect became. The study also examined colic, fussing
and crying and found no difference between the garlic and
placebo groups.

So, while certain babies may be sensitive to something in
their mothers' diet, on the whole there are more common
causes of infant crying.

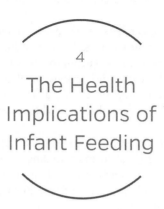

4

The Health Implications of Infant Feeding

Whether someone chooses to breastfeed or not, we have to acknowledge that human milk is what infants are biologically intended to consume. This means that research exploring the safety of alternative milks needs to compare the outcomes for infants fed this product to breastfed and breastmilk-fed babies. One way to do this is to explore rates of illness in babies who are partially or exclusively formula-fed, comparing the number of cases, duration and severity of illness with those recorded in breastfed infants.

Let's pick a random figure and say a breastfed baby has a 5 per cent chance of catching gastroenteritis in the first two years of life. We next need to know how many non-breastfed babies catch it during the same period, so let's pretend that we have a study that found the risk for a formula-fed infant was 20 per cent. Language that accurately described these findings would be 'Study suggests infants who aren't breastfed are at increased risk of gastroenteritis'.

When it comes to infant feeding, though, normal rules don't apply.

Instead the researchers or journalists reporting the story very often reverse the language. They use not-breastfeeding as the norm and compare the outcome of breastfed babies against that. The result is that the conclusion of the hypothetical study above would say 'breastfed babies at reduced risk of gastroenteritis'. The same happens when discussing severity and duration.

For example, a 2012 Unicef-funded report exploring the financial impact of formula feeding to the NHS didn't emphasise the burden artificial feeding places on the state. Instead we were told how much the NHS could save if more people breastfed:

> *A modest increase in breastfeeding rates would result in 21,000 fewer visits with babies to GPs for ear infections… In total it could save the NHS £40 million per year.*

This might not seem significant – it might feel to you, reading this, as though I'm being picky over wording – but as part of the big picture it's hugely important. Despite the fact that both statements in my first example seem to communicate the same information, we perceive and respond to the wording differently. Humans perceive things that 'carry risks' and those that 'carry benefits' in different ways.

In 2008 a working paper published by the Australian Centre for Economic Research on Health, entitled 'Voldemort and health professional knowledge of breastfeeding — do journal titles and abstracts accurately convey findings on differential health outcomes for formula fed infants?' examined 78 scientific studies cited by the American Academy of Pediatrics as evidence that breastfeeding is protective against a range of infectious and chronic diseases. The researchers discovered that a staggering 75 per cent of papers 'made no mention of artificial infant formula and would not challenge a reader's erroneous belief or assumption that artificial feeding carries no increased health risks for infants'. The paper's authors concluded:

> The AAP Policy Statement on breastfeeding and human milk stated that 'exclusive breastfeeding is the reference or normative model against which all alternative feeding methods must be measured with regard to growth, health, development and all other short- and long-term outcomes'.
>
> This approach can bias research through how the research hypothesis is specified, and through poor specification of infant feeding categories, with a tendency to underestimate the risk associated with non-human milk feeding.
>
> In recent years commentators have also highlighted the bias and negative effects on breastfeeding practices of normalising artificial feeding, referring for example, to 'the benefits of breastfeeding' rather than, for example, 'the risks of formula feeding'.
>
> Nevertheless, surveys reveal considerable cultural ambivalence and ignorance about the health consequences of artificial infant feeding. For example, some 30 per cent of mothers surveyed by the United States 'Babies Were Born To Be Breastfed!' campaign agreed with a statement that 'infant formula is as good as breastmilk', and only a minority of the survey population agreed that 'a breastfed baby is less likely to get ear infections or respiratory illness'.
>
> Likewise, a clear majority of public opinion in the United States supports the view that 'breastfeeding is healthier for babies', yet substantially more than half of

*the surveyed population disagree that 'feeding a baby
formula instead of breastmilk increases the chances the
baby will get sick'.*

When health professionals are making medical decisions,
how can they do so if they're not fully aware of risks?

We often hear it said that the evidence for breastfeeding
is not cut and dried. People claim that some studies show
breastfeeding 'has benefits,' but others don't, casting doubt on
the findings. Some argue that parental social status, education
and how much parents interact with the baby explain the
differences shown in studies. This is untrue; many studies
adjust for all these factors – but when we use benefit-based
language it's easy for confusion to arise.

Should we even be trying to prove that 'breast is best'? We
don't doubt that the milk of its own species is perfect for every
other living mammal on the planet.

The following is a non-exhaustive list of conditions that
several studies have suggested that non-breastfed babies may
be at increased risk of, sometimes with a direct dose-related
response depending on exclusivity and duration:

- Some childhood cancers before the age of 15
- Sudden infant death syndrome (SIDS)
- Breast cancer in later life
- IQ reduced by several points (particularly when baby
  carries a particular gene)
- Sickness and diarrhoea bugs including: gastroenteritis,
  E. coli and C. sakazakii (which can lead to meningitis)
- Crohn's disease and other inflammatory bowel disorders
- Both type 1 and 2 diabetes
- Low-birth-weight babies display reduced cognitive
  development
- Allergies

- Asthma
- Eczema
- Otitis media (ear infections)
- Respiratory tract infections
- Necrotising Enterocolitis (NEC)
- Bacterial meningitis
- Osteoporosis
- Obesity
- Pulmonary distress while feeding
- Ulcerative colitis (intestinal disorder)
- Suboptimal oral, dental and jaw development
- Constipation and digestion problems
- High cholesterol in later life
- Urinary tract infections
- Higher blood pressure in childhood and later life
- Atherosclerosis (plaque build-up inside arteries)
- Coeliac disease (gluten intolerance)

Not breastfeeding has been linked to increased risk to the mother of:

- Breast cancer
- Post-partum haemorrhage
- Ovarian cancer
- Endometrial cancer
- Rheumatoid arthritis
- Osteoporosis
- Cardiovascular problems
- Postnatal depression
- Type 2 diabetes
- Anaemia (iron deficiency)

Another way to explore the health implications of feeding method is by looking at the make-up of breastmilk. Many are surprised to hear that breastmilk contains hundreds of constituents that can't be replicated in formula, with more regularly being identified as science advances. As we begin to understand the role each plays and how they interact, we can use this alongside the outcome-based evidence discussed above.

Let's take for example the thymus gland, a small organ that sits just beneath the breastbone. It's an unusual one as it grows in size and activity until puberty and then begins to shrink and reduce activity until it's replaced entirely by fat and connective tissue. Removal in adulthood doesn't appear to cause serious problems, whereas its absence in infancy can significantly hinder the appropriate development of the immune system. There's still a lot to learn about the thymus. Immunologists Kelley et al have noted:

> The involution (shrinkage) of the thymus gland is one of the cardinal bio-markers of ageing, with some suggesting the subsequent decline of thymic hormones gradually robs the body of its ability to fight off infectious diseases, autoimmune diseases, and cancer.

What is known, however, is that the work done by the thymus prior to it shrinking has a lifelong impact. The thymus serves:
- To trap immature stem cells from bone marrow and circulating blood.
- To pre-process these cells, enabling them to become capable of maturing into T-cells, a type of lymphocyte or white blood cell that plays an important role in the immune system.

These T-cells migrate through the body and serve a number of functions:
- Some disrupt harmful bacteria.

- Some are involved in recognising 'foreignness' and assisting a second sub-population of white blood cells from the bone marrow to respond.
- Some seed lymph nodes (which act as filters or traps for foreign particles) and lymphatic tissue (connective tissue that contains large numbers of white blood cells).

T-cells are essential to the regulation of immune responses. Research suggests that non-exclusively breastfed infants have reduced thymic function. A paper found that:

At 4 months the geometric mean thymic index was 38.3 in exclusively breastfed infants, 27.3 in partially breastfed infants and 18.3 in formula fed infants. This finding was independent of weight, length, sex and previous or current illness. There was no significant difference in mean thymic index at birth between the three feeding groups and mean thymic index had increased in all three groups from birth to 4 months.

The authors concluded:

For the formula-fed infants it seems that the thymus remains large for a period and then decreases in size after breastfeeding has been terminated. The thymus is considerably larger in breastfed than in formula-fed infants at the age of 4 months. The above data indicates the thymus is less than half the size in an exclusively formula fed infant.

Another paper found:

At 10 months the thymic index was significantly higher in those still being breastfed compared to infants who had stopped breast-feeding between 8 and 10 months of age (P=0.05). This difference became more significant when controlled for the influence of infectious diseases (P=0.03). In infants still breastfed at 10 months there was a significant correlation between the number of breastfeeds per day and their thymic index. (P=0.01)

We know that breastmilk contains a constituent called interleukin 7 (IL-7), a growth factor secreted by cells in bone marrow and the thymus. This growth factor is critical in the development of T-cells and researchers confirmed that it could explain the difference in the resulting thymus size and efficiency, adding: 'These data suggest possible implications for long-term programming of immunity.'

A 2011 study exploring the topic further concluded:

Our study provides direct evidence that interleukin 7, a factor which is critical in the development of T lymphocytes, when maternally derived can transfer across the intestine of the offspring, increase T cell production in the thymus and support the survival of T cells in the peripheral secondary lymphoid tissue.

In short, the IL-7 in breastmilk transfers to the baby, survives in his body, increases his own T-cell production and then supports his survival.

Next let's look at pertussis, or whooping cough. Although research repeatedly shows that babies who are not breastfed suffer at a higher rate than those who are, this is dismissed by many (including doctors and other health professionals) as coincidental or insignificant.

In 1989 a study found that breastmilk contained significant amounts of two different types of pertussis-specific antibodies.

Another study that tested women (in an area where many were found to be immune from natural exposure), discovered that 87 per cent produced pertussis antibodies in their colostrum. A 2010 study found colostrum samples showed a 100 per cent average transfer rate of one type of antibody (those that are the same as passed via the placenta), and variable levels of another type depending on the degree of exposure that each mother had to several antigens. Overall high antibody levels demonstrated a high rate of protection, while lower levels weren't as reliable. Researchers concluded:

> *Our data demonstrated the effectiveness of anti-pertussis antibodies in bacterial pathogenesis neutralization, emphasizing the importance of placental transfer and breast-feeding in protecting infants against respiratory infections caused by Bordetella pertussis.*

What about mums vaccinated during pregnancy?
Research suggests that vaccinating mum during pregnancy increases the levels of both types of antibodies in her breastmilk; what's more, unlike the more rapidly waning antibodies passed via the placenta, they're not short-lived:

> *Interestingly, antenatal maternal vaccination appears to positively influence the production of specific antibodies transferred to the infant via breast milk for at least 5–6 months postpartum.*

But it gets even more interesting than just antibodies. The 2010 study mentioned above concluded:

> *Bacterial neutralization may not be solely because of the functional activity of specific antibodies, and suggests*

that other anti-infective factors present in human serum and colostrum may contribute to non-specific bacterial neutralization. Several non-specific anti-infective components capable of inhibiting bacterial pathogenesis have been found in human milk.

A 2015 paper published in the *Journal of Vaccines & Vaccination* reads:

The dawn of maternal vaccination is an important milestone in breastmilk immunity. Breastmilk per se has immunopotential that protects the infant from important childhood diseases both in the immediate neonatal period and in the long term. Its immune nutritive attributes confer this exclusive early nourishment a cutting edge in defence that no other human nutrient can yet offer.

The immunological components in breastmilk are many. They are diverse and multifunctional. It is proposed that vaccines that are given to the mother can pass through breastmilk and potentially utilise these breastmilk components to augment action and protection.

The increasing global incidence of antibiotic resistance to treat important infections affecting the infant makes it crucial to emphasize the importance of breastfeeding and possibly enhancing microbial protection transferred through maternal vaccination as a primary preventive strategy.

The authors conclude that more antenatal clinics should routinely practise the delivery of this multi-pronged system, as 'primary disease prevention is achieved both by breastfeeding and by vaccination'.

We'd need an entire book to explore every illness and

every constituent of breastmilk. There are proteins that can cause cell suicide in numerous types of cancer cells, and stem cells that can develop into different cells in the body, serving as an internal repair system. Lymphocytes kill infected cells directly, or mobilise other components of the immune system. There are enzymes and antibodies that actively seek out and destroy harmful pathogens, sweeping them from the body and regulating immune response. Anti-infective factors, hormones, growth factors, anti-inflammatories and more are present.

A 2015 study states:

> In the majority of freshly expressed breast milk samples, >90% of total milk cells are viable. It can be estimated that human milk contains 200–260,000 leukocytes/m (a white blood cell involved in counteracting foreign substances and disease); and that normally breastfed infants receive 94,000–351 million leukocytes from breast milk on a daily basis, of which >90% are viable and can exert immunomodulatory functions. During periods of infection of either the mother or the infant, the number of leukocytes ingested daily by breastfed infants can reach the billions. Studies so far indicate that maternal breast milk–derived leukocytes provide active immunity to the infant, both assisting the development of its own immune system and fighting pathogens directly.
>
> It will be of interest to examine whether the immune system and health of infants fed formula, which does not include any viable cells, are in any way compromised specifically by the lack of maternal breast milk leukocytic support in the short- and/or long term compared with infants fed fresh breast milk. Previous studies have investigated the immune function of breastfed vs. formula-fed infants and have evidently shown higher

infection rates in infants fed formula than in those fed breast milk.

I know it can be uncomfortable to talk about the risks of different feeding methods. Sometimes in a community setting health differences can be difficult to see; plenty of mums know breastfed babies who have suffered health problems, and formula-fed infants who are fine. It's only when data relating to large numbers of babies are collated that visible patterns of risk emerge.

It's also important to remember that we are talking about risks and not absolutes. Breastfeeding is not a guarantee a baby won't become sick, and formula does not guarantee they will. We also have to look beyond babyhood into childhood and adulthood and consider long-term outcomes. We need to remember that in the big picture of gut microbiome, what happens before and after milk feeding – in terms of nutrition, medications and the bacterial population that thrives as a result – is also likely to contribute significantly to overall health.

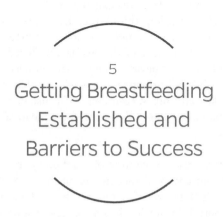

5

Getting Breastfeeding Established and Barriers to Success

Many people seem to believe that the ability to breastfeed (or not) is random; if you're lucky it works, but a lot can't do it. Over the years I've heard many reasons for women's inability to breastfeed, including: fair hair, red hair, pale and sensitive skin, a low pain threshold, nipples that are too flat/big/pointy/droopy, not eating the right food or not making milk of the right quality.

In fact, lactation is a pretty sound science. Of course there are always variances, because human bodies aren't always entirely predictable, but on the whole the mechanism of what makes a painless feed with effective milk transfer is thoroughly understood.

We also know that birth and what happens immediately afterwards has an impact on how easy it is for mum and baby to establish breastfeeding. Long labours, very rapid deliveries, assisted deliveries, caesarean sections, even a rapid pushing stage – can make some babies a bit stiffer and fussier or sleepier in the first few days or weeks, sometimes making feeding a little more challenging.

There are some key things that have been shown to hinder or help when it comes to establishing breastfeeding. Sometimes one or more of the risk factors listed below is unavoidable or unachievable due to medical necessity; this does *not* mean that breastfeeding won't work. Some babies will still take to the breast easily, but it can also be reassuring for some parents to know it's normal for some to take a little more time.

1. Risk factor: early separation of mum and baby

Keeping mum and baby together as much as possible after birth can help things get off to the best start. A typical healthy, term newborn is born with the reflexes and instincts to feed, and will start spontaneously sucking and rooting around 15–20 minutes after birth. He will then gradually start shifting towards the breast, using the scent and taste on his hands and mum's body to assist his journey, which is often known as the 'breast crawl'. Some babies do this quite rapidly, but it's also normal for this process to take up to an hour or even longer – even after an uncomplicated vaginal delivery.

Evidence suggests that disturbing mum and baby during this period can result in baby becoming more 'disorganised' when she returns to the breast for that first feed. This means she may find it harder to coordinate finding the breast and latching on effectively. If mum is recovering from surgery or needs other medical attention, placing baby skin-to-skin with the second parent or another family member or friend is the next best thing until mum is ready.

It's common for separation to occur for routine things like weighing the baby, or dressing them quickly, and sometimes baby is washed, which removes the smells that can help baby navigate to the breast. Mums who have caesarean sections often tell us it's very important that they don't return from theatre to find baby dressed; they need time for skin-to-skin and to 'discover' their newborn – whether in recovery or hours later. Parents need to know that they can ask their caregivers to wait before carrying out any routine procedures.

2. Protect factor: let the baby initiate feeding where possible

As discussed above babies run through a sequence of behaviours before feeding that include rooting and looking at the mother's face. A 'crawling phase', followed by licking, sucking and then sleeping follows, and research has shown that allowing the baby to transition through all these phases results in optimal early self-regulation: in other words, the best chance of a good breastfeed.

If mum is comfortably reclined (at around 45 degrees so she can see her baby easily is better than being flat, unless there's a medical reason), with baby on her chest, baby can rest his feet on her and push against her. Babies are born with a walking or stepping reflex that persists until around two months of age; when baby's feet touch a surface, she will lift one foot and then the other (which looks like walking). If mum naturally supports her baby in this position across his shoulders, he will begin gravitating towards the breast. He navigates his way using a combination of sight, scent and taste; mum's breasts smell like amniotic fluid to help guide him, and her nipples have darkened in pregnancy as a visual cue. Baby then typically grasps the nipple with a hand, then swap this for their mouth.

3. Risk factor: opiates, particularly close to the time of delivery

Pain medications such as pethidine and meptid cross the placenta and have been shown to have the potential to make babies sleepy and uncoordinated, particularly when they are born shortly after the drugs have been given. Many midwives suggest they're more appropriately used to allow mum to sleep during a very long labour, when she is likely to have a good amount of time left before she delivers.

4. Protect factor: avoid teats

Bottle feeding requires a different action with the mouth, lips and tongue, and so some compare trying to learn to use both breast and bottle simultaneously to being given either chopsticks or a knife and fork alternately at each feed, when you've no prior experience of using either. Add to this a newborn's undeveloped cognitive ability and reflex and instinct-driven behaviours, and it's easy to see why babies may try out some of the techniques that work on the bottle at the breast, which can lead to problems breastfeeding.

5. Risk factor: baby not latching or feeding, and impact on milk supply

This may be due to prematurity, illness, a difficult birth or something like a significant tongue tie that prevents baby from extending their tongue to grasp the breast.

6. Protect factor: expressing

Mums wanting to breastfeed should be encouraged to express as soon as possible after birth if the baby is unable to latch, or attach effectively to transfer colostrum. Learning about hand expression techniques and different breast pump options before baby arrives can be beneficial if you later find yourself needing to supplement some extra milk. (See chapter 8.)

7. Risk factor: unwanted hands-on breastfeeding support

Nobody should grab mum's breast or push baby's head on to the breast when helping to latch on. Nobody should even consider touching a mum, her breast or her baby without her explicit consent. In the vast majority of circumstances mums can be helped without being touched. I think this is really important to stress, as some mums may delay seeking support if they feel uncomfortable with the thought that someone may touch them.

Pushing on baby's head can also trigger a hostile response in baby, causing them to jerk their head backwards to resist. It can also cause baby to be sensitive to any touch to his head when feeding, particularly if he's stiff or sore anyway following delivery. Would you like it if I pushed your head into your dinner?

Parents should be encouraged to have the confidence to stop any behaviour they do not feel 100 per cent happy with. A simple 'stop' can bring an immediate halt when the situation requires, combined with raising a hand if necessary to put up a physical barrier. Parents can then request more information about what the person is doing and why, or simply decline physical contact entirely.

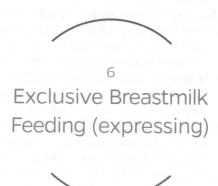

6

Exclusive Breastmilk Feeding (expressing)

Some mothers feed their babies only breastmilk, but instead of feeding directly from the breast they express (using a pump, or by hand) and then feed the milk back to the baby. Mums might want to do this for any number of reasons, and while it's often just for a short period, some continue to exclusively express for months.

Many parents I see are unaware that it's possible to maintain a breastmilk supply by pumping alone. While it definitely isn't an easy option, it is the best option for some families.

In order to maintain her supply, in the early days a mum needs to express as frequently as a baby would feed, which is 8–12 times per 24 hours. For a typical new mum 8 or 9 times is usually sufficient, but a mum who has previously experienced supply problems, or has other concerns such as reduced glandular tissue, would aim for more. This can seem daunting at first, particularly for first-time parents, but the reality is that feeding a young baby is a 24-hour job however you do it.

If a mum is trying to fit in expressing sessions, there are

different ways to achieve the number she needs. Expressing sessions don't have to be at perfectly-spaced intervals, such as every two or three hours around the clock; some mums pump frequently during the day, with slightly longer gaps in the evening, and pump once overnight. They would then have a longer gap before another expressing session in the early morning. (After all, babies feeding directly from the breast have very varied feeding patterns.) Breastfeeding hormones peak in the early hours of the morning, so for most women one expressing session during this time is crucial to effectively maintain a full milk supply. This is particularly true in the early weeks and for some women in the longer term too.

One study found that mums who expressed when they woke naturally when their baby roused obtained more milk than when they expressed to set patterns determined by a clock and alarm. This assumes that your baby self-rouses every few hours; some babies are sleepier, particularly if they are jaundiced, and if this is the case your healthcare provider will usually suggest an alarm to wake you at regular intervals.

Once milk volumes increase, it's recommended that mum expresses approximately as frequently as baby feeds. It's a really common mistake to underestimate a baby's longer-term needs based on the first few days of life. What can happen is that when milk is suddenly abundant, mum can pump a large amount of milk compared to the initial colostrum. After four or five sessions she may have collected all she needs for that particular day. It can be tempting then for a tired mum to head off to bed for a long stretch of unbroken sleep (because someone else can feed the expressed milk), without realising that an abnormally long period without milk removal can slow down her production – and the next day the baby's needs will have increased.

As baby gets older, many mums find they can express less often and still obtain the same volumes – just like an older baby might start to feed a bit less frequently. Some mums of five and six-month-olds can get all the milk needed in four or five sessions, while others find more pumping sessions are needed to result in enough milk for all feeds.

The biggest barriers to exclusive expressing are time and practicalities. As the baby gets a little older, finding the extra time to pump and clean equipment on top of actually feeding the milk can become more challenging.

As with all parenting, mums who express often learn tips and tricks to help them manage their time most effectively. This could be something practical like taking a cool box upstairs at night so they don't need to come downstairs, or working out the best time during the day to express to obtain the most volume.

Why exclusive breastmilk feeding?

Worldwide, health authorities recommend six months of exclusive breastmilk feeding for babies. This means no water, other milk or food. The gut of a baby who has only received breastmilk is particularly unique and is sometimes referred to as a 'virgin gut'.

Many people have now heard of 'good bacteria' and 'bad bacteria' (which we kill with antibiotics), but these terms are overly simplistic. Bacteria are complicated and a single strain may both help and hinder human health. However, everyone's gut contains trillions of bacteria, with a huge spectrum of different species. As in any ecosystem, some organisms keep others in check, preventing those linked with yeasts, inflammation, illness or disease from taking over. This intestinal microflora, which used to be called 'gut flora', is now known as the gut microbiota, or the gut microbiome.

The microbiome is thought to act almost like a second brain in the gut, and is intrinsically linked to many other functions in the body. It helps to stimulate the digestive process and aids the absorption of nutrients. It assists in producing vitamins including B and K, and it has a role in training the immune system to respond only to pathogens, regulating weight, inflammation levels and metabolism. In short, the gut microbiota has a continuous and dynamic effect on the gut and systemic immune system.

Numerous studies have identified differences between the microbiome of babies who are exclusively breastfed, those who receive some breastmilk and those who are exclusively formula fed. Unsurprisingly, changes in the gut are most serious for those babies that are most vulnerable – premature infants.

In the 1970s, the relationship between feeding method and a disease called necrotising enterocolitis (NEC) was first identified. It's the most common and devastating disease in premature newborns, and has proved one of the most difficult to eradicate, making it a priority for research.

A multi-centre trial demonstrated the protective effect of breastmilk in the fight against NEC. The lowest incidence, at 1.2 per cent, was in the group given only breastmilk, compared with 7.2 per cent in the group that was exclusively formula-fed. Among babies born at more than 30 weeks' gestation, NEC was rare in those whose diet included any breast milk; it was 20 times more common in those fed only formula. In fact, the authors concluded:

With the fall in the use of breast milk in British neonatal units, exclusive formula feeding could account for an estimated 500 extra cases of necrotising enterocolitis each year. About 100 of these infants would die.

Researchers have identified a specific epidermal growth factor (EGF) that occurs in breastmilk as being important in preventing NEC. One might think that as a result of this knowledge it would have become a priority to ensure that as many premature infants as possible have access to human milk; be that from their own mother or a breastmilk bank that stores and pasteurises milk other mothers have donated.

Alas, not: research is under way that aims to genetically modify soybeans to produce EGF, which will then be used to create a specialist infant formula. Since breastmilk is free, there is no profit to be made – but the potential profits from an 'anti-NEC formula' are enormous.

Of course, many babies are not at risk of NEC. However, we shouldn't assume that the gut changes in formula-fed healthy newborns are insignificant.

A baby is born with some pre-exposure to mum's bacteria, both from the placenta and via the birth canal during delivery. What happens next dictates which bacteria are most likely to become established in the baby's gut microbiome.

If a baby receives colostrum and then breastmilk, which contain both good bacteria (probiotics), and the food to help these good bacteria set up residence and thrive (prebiotics), we know that interesting things happen and a unique environment dominated by good bacteria develops. Acidity levels are key to this, and pH is important for understanding the differences between the guts of breastfed and non-breastfed babies.

The pH scale is a measure of whether something is acid or alkali. It runs from 0 to 14, with 7 being neutral. If a pH value is below 7 it is acid; if it is above 7 it's alkaline. In exclusively breastfed term babies, gut acidity levels are around pH 5.1–5.4, which is acidic. Many good bacteria thrive in an acidic environment; in fact they produce acids to help create the ideal conditions to multiply. The more good bacteria you have, the less likely it is that an odd harmful pathogen will survive or grow to the extent that it causes harm.

These harmful pathogens multiply better in a neutral or alkaline environment. *Staphylococci, Streptococci, H. influenzae* and *Meningococcus* all proliferate more successfully in alkaline conditions. If babies don't receive human milk, it is much less certain which bacteria will establish a foothold. The gut acidity levels of an exclusively formula-fed baby vary widely, from slightly less acidic at 5.9, right up to an alkaline 7.3.

This might not sound like a huge shift, but each whole pH value is *ten times* more acidic than the next highest value. So pH 5 is ten times more acidic than pH 6, and 100 times (10 times 10) more acidic than pH 7. So in some cases the formula-fed baby's gut is 100 times less acidic than that of a breastfed baby (pH 7.3 compared to pH 5.1)

In this context, preventing NEC is likely to mean considering the whole gut environment, not one specific growth factor. Studies suggest that in premature infants, medications which inhibit acid secretion (including some medications prescribed for acid reflux) are associated with increased incidence of both NEC and other infections.

Thus, researchers decided to test whether they could create the opposite effect by acidifying premature infant formula:

> It appears that acidifying the feedings of small premature infants to a pH low enough to inhibit bacterial proliferation in the stomach significantly lowers the risk of necrotizing enterocolitis.

Or we could just give them breastmilk.

We don't yet know the long-term implications of gut acidity imbalance for either term or premature babies, as there's still so much research to do.

When babies are fed a mixture of breastmilk and formula supplements, the mean gut pH is approximately 5.7–6.0

during the first four weeks, falling to 5.45 by the sixth week. This means that in the first six weeks a mix-fed baby has a gut that is 2–8 times less acidic than a baby receiving solely breastmilk. By six weeks acidity levels are more comparable, although the bacterial profiles still differ.

Another factor to consider is the spaces between the cells in a baby's gut at birth. These allow the thousands of active constituents in breastmilk to move directly into the baby's bloodstream. However, if the baby does not receive breastmilk, potentially harmful pathogens and allergens in formula milk have an easy access point too. Evidence suggests that when breastfeeding starts immediately after birth, rapid closure of the gut happens in the first few days of life, although it takes weeks for the junctions to fully mature and tighten. A delay of 24 hours before breastfeeding, or the use of infant formula, appears to delay this early closure, and by seven days breastfed babies have significantly tighter cell spacing than those fed either regular or hypoallergenic formula.

Risk of insufficient intake

The above is clearly an argument in favour of babies not receiving formula milk, and it demonstrates that there are health implications for babies if they do not receive breastmilk. However, there are also very real risks of not having enough to eat and drink, which should make us wary of overstating the case for exclusive breastmilk feeding in our current system that lacks universal access to donor human milk and high-quality breastfeeding support. In the short term newborns are at risk of dehydration, which can have neurological consequences and potentially result in organ failure. Newborns can go rapidly from absolutely fine at birth to an extremely worrying position in just a few days if they can't transfer milk.

In the longer term, babies who have extremely slow

or faltering growth may not receive enough vitamins and minerals; they may have reduced energy levels and start to sleep for abnormally long periods at night (seeming settled and not hungry). Some babies will protest loudly that they can't quite transfer enough milk, or will stay at the breast for long periods, protesting if they're moved from their food source. Others don't protest about their reduced intake, perhaps because protesting takes energy they're trying to conserve. A confident healthcare provider should be able to discuss the risks and benefits of different plans, but as an International Board Certified Lactation Consultant (IBCLC) the first rule is always 'feed the baby'.

Antibodies

As adults we make antibodies when we come into contact with disease-causing microbes. One type, called SIgA, (which adults make in abundance) is particularly important, as infants are completely unable to produce their own for the first two months of life, and by one year of age they still only produce around 20 per cent of adult levels. Yet SIgA serves as the first line of defence in protecting the gut from toxins and harmful microbes, and is so important that it's sometimes referred to as 'antiseptic paint'. This antibody is not only directly absorbed into the baby's bloodstream in the first 18–24 hours of life when they receive colostrum, but after that works by coating the digestive tract, making it sticky. What it does next is nothing short of brilliant.

Through a process known as 'immune exclusion', SIgA seals the spaces between the cells of the gut, effectively blocking the receptors that harmful bacteria attach to in order to become established. It then attaches itself to the problem bacteria and entraps them in mucous, so they can be destroyed. What's clever is that SIgA ignores bacteria that aren't harmful, and appears to let 'helpful constituents' through. SIgA has been shown to assist in clearing pathogens of dietary, bacterial and viral origin, and it also directly influences the baby's gut microbiota and balance of bacteria. More recently researchers have also identified that it has the ability to regulate autoimmune disease, although further research is needed in this area.

Some very interesting work highlights the consequences for mice pups which do not receive SIgA and cannot produce their own. Mice are used because their 'genetic, biological and behaviour characteristics closely resemble those of humans, and many symptoms of human conditions can be replicated in mice and rats'. The pups that grew up without SIgA had different communities of gut bacteria, and had more of certain groups that are found in the guts of humans suffering inflammatory bowel disease. These early changes persisted into adulthood and left the mice permanently susceptible to inflammation, even if they could eventually make SIgA for themselves.

Additionally, in mice – as in humans – gut microbes interact with other cells to create a sealed barrier, keeping foreign material out of the deeper intestinal tissue. In the mice pups without SIgA, bacteria were able to pass into the underlying lymph nodes. One of the study authors said:

> These lymph nodes should be absolutely sterile. When you take them out of an adult mouse and culture them, you'll find no bacteria. When we took lymph nodes from offspring who didn't get SIgA in their milk, they were loaded with bacteria.

What does this mean? The lymphatic system is complex, but can be simply described as a network of thin tubes and nodes that make and move lymph (a clear or white fluid) from tissues to the bloodstream. Unfiltered lymph is carried to nodes, which act like a biological filtering system. They make cells to help fight any infection, and filter the fluid to remove foreign material such as bacteria and damaged or cancerous cells, before the cleaned fluid is carried away round the system.

When you have an infection and can feel swollen glands in your neck, armpit or groin, this comes from bacteria trapped in nodes. Cells that line the walls of the lymph nodes work to destroy these bacteria and the swelling and pain subside. The researchers reported:

> *The most abundant species [found in the lymph nodes] was Ochrobactrum anthropi – an opportunistic bacterium that's been linked to a growing number of infections in hospital patients.*

The researchers also showed that these mice could then pass on different microbes to their own offspring when the time came for them to produce milk, potentially leading to further consequences in the next generation.

What else do we know?
- Older research has shown that relatively small amounts of formula (one supplement per 24 hours) will damage the SIgA barrier, and result in a shift in the microbiome to more closely resemble that of a formula-fed baby, becoming almost indistinguishable from normal adult flora within 24 hours. Very old research (1932) suggests it would take 2–4 weeks of exclusive breastfeeding to return the gut to a comparable state.
- Breastfed babies can be sensitised to cow's milk protein by the giving of just one bottle in the first three days of life. If a supplement is needed during this time and breastmilk isn't available, hypoallergenic formula may be preferred.

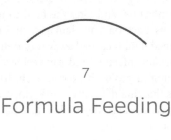

7

Formula Feeding

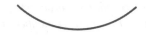

Rates of formula feeding

British babies drink a lot of formula milk. We know this because every five years the government used to commission an Infant Feeding Survey designed to take a snapshot of infant feeding practices in the UK, but this has now been cancelled and didn't take place in 2015. In the most recent study, published in 2012, we learn that:

At birth
- 81% of babies are put to the breast at least once, or given one or more feeds of expressed milk
- 69% are exclusively breast or breastmilk fed
- 19% are exclusively formula fed

By 1 week
- 45% of babies are exclusively breast or breastmilk fed
- 31% are exclusively formula fed
- 24% are receiving a mix of both

By 6 weeks
- 45% are exclusively formula fed
- 32% are receiving a mix of both
- 23% of babies are exclusively breast or breastmilk fed

By 12 weeks
- 83% are either exclusively formula fed, receiving a mix of both, or are also taking solids
- 17% babies are exclusively breast or breastmilk fed

By 4 months
- 88% are either exclusively formula fed, receiving a mix of both, or are also taking solids
- 12% are still breastfeeding exclusively

By 6 months
- 34% are still receiving any breastmilk
- 1% are exclusively breast or breastmilk fed

Furthermore
- Around three in ten mothers had experienced some kind of feeding problem, either in the hospital, birth centre or unit (29%), or in the early weeks after leaving (30%).
- 90% of mothers who stopped breastfeeding in the first few days and weeks said they would have liked to continue.
- Just under half of mothers breastfeeding in the hospital, birth centre or unit (48%) were informed about how to recognise that their baby was getting enough milk.

If over half of new mums are unsure how to tell their baby is getting enough milk, and so many mothers feel that they have to stop breastfeeding earlier than they wanted, we clearly need more and better breastfeeding support. However, we also need to consider that if so many babies are getting so much formula milk, it's imperative that parents have good information about how to use it as safely as possible.

Preparing formula safely

Most formula milks today are made from cow's milk, not because this is close to human milk (on the contrary, unprocessed dairy is unsuitable for human infants), but because cows are easy to keep and milk, producing good volumes in relation to the costs of keeping them. Historically, formula milks resolved the problem of what to do with the whey that remained from cheese-making. Once discarded as a waste product, it could now be marketed and sold.

Incredible as it may seem, it remains impossible to directly compare infant formula milks and make a choice as to which is the best. Infant formula in the UK is regulated by the Infant Formula Act. Under the provisions of the law, manufacturers are not required to fully disclose the ingredients in their products – so they don't. While the packaging must list the nutritional composition, the basic ingredients that those components are derived from are not required. So only the formula companies themselves know whether their additives are derived from egg, algae, fish or other ingredients. (For much more information see the resources on the First Steps Nutrition website www. firststepsnutrition.org)

It's also important to remember that powdered formula isn't sterile; there are risks of contamination all the way through the process, from the raw ingredients, through production after pasteurisation and then in the reformulation or in the can at home. The biggest risks are from *Cronobacter sakazakii* (previously called *Enterobacter sakazakii*) and *Salmonella*. In 2005 researchers found that 0 to 12 per cent of samples they tested were contaminated, using milk from five different companies; a 2010 study found 9 out of 149 samples were contaminated with *E. sakazakii*.

Infection with *Cronobacter sakazakii* may be rare, but it can be extremely nasty, and there are strong links with meningitis, septicemia and NEC. In reported outbreaks, typically over 50 per cent of infants have died, while many who survive suffer severe lasting complications including neurological disorders. Formula powder is dry and provides the perfect environment for bacteria to grow and thrive, and in 50–80 per cent of cases powdered infant formula is both the vehicle and the source (direct or indirect) of *Cronobacter*-induced illness.

This may sound dramatic or scary – but the key thing to remember is that the risk can be dramatically reduced by taking steps to make up and store formula safely. Using boiled water cooled to no less than 70 degrees centigrade significantly reduces the levels of bacteria in prepared formula. Discarding any leftover formula within an hour prevents any remaining pathogens from increasing in number again, a risk that increases further once baby's saliva has entered the mix. This is really important as, in the above-mentioned study, 8 of the 9 cases of contamination showed low numbers of *Cronobacter*, meaning that mixing the powder with water of an adequate temperature and using it immediately should reduce the risk of infection to a minimal level.

Full guidelines on safer formula preparation from the NHS choices website

Step 1: Fill the kettle with at least 1 litre of fresh tap water from the cold tap (don't use water that has been boiled before).

Step 2: Boil the water. Then leave the water to cool in the kettle for no more than 30 minutes so that it remains at a temperature of at least 70°C. (NB – please check this using your own equipment, as my experiments at home found some kettles don't hit boiling point and all retain heat differently. In some kettles the water hit 70 after less than 20 minutes, and was significantly cooler than 70°C after half an hour)

Step 3: Clean and disinfect the surface you are going to use.

Step 4: It's really important that you WASH YOUR HANDS.

Step 5: If you are using a cold-water steriliser, shake off any excess solution from the bottle and the teat, or rinse the bottle with cooled boiled water from the kettle (not the tap).

Step 6: Stand the bottle on a clean surface.

Step 7: Keep the teat and cap on the upturned lid of the steriliser. Avoid putting them on the work surface.

Step 8: Follow the manufacturer's instructions and pour the correct amount of water into the bottle. Double-check that the water level is correct.

Step 9: Loosely fill the scoop with formula – according to the manufacturer's instructions – and level it off using either the flat edge of a clean, dry knife or the leveller provided.

Step 10: Holding the edge of the teat, put it on the bottle. Then screw the retaining ring on to the bottle.

Step 11: Cover the teat with the cap and shake the bottle until the powder is dissolved.

Step 12: It is important to cool the formula so it is not too hot to drink. Do this by holding the bottom half of the bottle under cold running water. Move the bottle about under the tap to ensure even cooling. Make sure that the water does not touch the cap covering the teat.

Step 13: Test the temperature of the infant formula on the inside of your wrist before giving it to your baby. It should be body temperature, which means it should feel warm or cool, but not hot.

Step 14: If there is any made-up infant formula left after a feed, throw it away.

Not surprisingly, some parents find this guidance a little overwhelming when they have a new baby, and may, at least initially, want an alternative (discussed below). If parents don't have the facilities to prepare the feed at the time it's needed, and have no alternative but to make bottles in advance, cooling and refrigerating immediately is recommended.

Ready-to-feed formula (RTF)

Bottles of liquid formula are sterile, and can be kept for up to 48 hours in the fridge if chilled immediately. Following a 2012 study highlighting the risks associated with *Cronobacter*, some authorities now recommend ready-to-feed formula for all formula-fed babies until three months of age.

A significant barrier to long-term use of RTF formula is the cost compared to powdered infant formula.

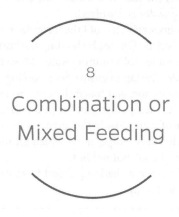

8

Combination or Mixed Feeding

Mixed feeding, sometimes known as combination feeding, means that a baby is either breastfeeding or receiving expressed milk as well as formula, either as a short-term measure or a long-term plan.

As we know that formula supplements cause changes in the gut of a breastfed baby, some parents wonder whether it is worth continuing to give breastmilk if you've decided to introduce some formula. We've already mentioned that there are thousands of constituents of breastmilk. Even one feed per day is considered beneficial for baby's immune system. And beyond nutrition, all the other reasons to breastfeed that we discussed in chapter 1 still apply.

Is supplementation a slippery slope?

How mixed feeding impacts on breastfeeding and milk supply depends on many different factors, because each mum and baby pair is unique. People can tell you what happened to them in a similar situation, or recount what the books say, but there may be subtle differences in the circumstances, mum's body, baby and so on.

If a mum is exclusively breastfeeding well, has a typical milk supply, her baby is thriving and she chooses to replace a breastfeed with a bottle of formula, her body gets the signal that milk wasn't needed. If this is a one-off, or she regularly intends to replace that feed, it may cause no further problems for that mum; her supply may be 'bulletproof' and long gaps between feeds, or missed feeds, may cause no noticeable problems, particularly in the short-term.

Another mum in the same situation, whose milk supply was just being maintained by the feeds she was doing, might find that replacing even one feed could cause a noticeable reduction in how much milk she produces. If this happens, more formula supplement is used to cover the shortfall, and so she can gradually find herself moving in an unplanned direction.

Of course there are lots of shades of grey too – some mums might find they can miss one feed without problems, yet two results in baby feeding much more frequently to increase supply again – it's really individual to each dyad.

Sometimes babies simply aren't feeding well enough to transfer enough milk at the breast. In this situation, formula can be used as a 'stepping stone'. In this case a supplement of formula isn't likely to directly impact on mum's supply, any more than the lack of milk removal by the baby was. Her breasts are already receiving the message that the milk isn't needed, which as we know reduces production. The baby, however, is receiving additional milk they otherwise wouldn't have obtained, which can give them energy to then feed better from the breast.

Breastfeeding workers need to be skilled enough to identify exactly when and to what level support is required – without undermining mum's supply or leaving baby without adequate nutrition. The 'ideal', in cases where babies are struggling a little, is that problems are identified early. If the problem is picked up soon after birth, when milk volumes first increase, ensuring regular and effective milk removal can protect mum's supply and provide any supplements needed for baby. If mum doesn't get early help and struggles on for weeks or months, by the time the problem is found supply may have reduced, meaning that additional milk, either donated breastmilk or formula, is needed to 'top up'. Mum can then work to increase supply again, but rebuilding a supply is more work than maintaining it.

The biggest risk of supplementation leading to an end to breastfeeding comes when support is lacking. Parents have no idea why their baby won't gain weight, despite seemingly feeding lots, or not seeming to settle for long before he's signaling he wants to feed again. The transition can be anything from an extremely rapid swap to formula (from that point on), or a gradual switch as more and more is given as supply reduces.

Often mums and babies just need a tweak to increase the amount of breastmilk baby receives, but if nobody knows how to help then unnecessary formula use may be the result.

What equipment is best for mixed feeding?
In the first six weeks of life the standard guidance for breastfeeding mothers is to try and avoid bottles. There is debate about whether 'nipple confusion' exists, and I think that's probably because there isn't a 'one size fits all' answer. A baby who has already mastered the skill of breastfeeding well is less likely to have problems transitioning between a breast and a bottle than a baby that is struggling to breastfeed.

The babies that pose the biggest dilemma are those who are struggling to transfer enough milk to remain hydrated or grow well. Clearly there is sometimes a need to supplement with extra milk, but these babies, in my experience, are also those who are more at risk of preferring the faster flow of a bottle.

It's logical really, as babies are pretty well programmed for survival – think about what you would do if you were hungry and could get an easy hit from a bottle rather than working hard at the breast. Contrary to popular belief, breastfeeding isn't 'hard work' for a baby if it's all going well, but if latch is shallow or mum's supply is low it can become so. Is it any surprise that these babies won't tolerate a long session at the breast if the milk isn't flowing?

Tiny babies younger than a few weeks are more prone to have problems switching between breast and bottle. I've witnessed hungry babies fall asleep as soon as they latch to the breast, or who don't stir when a nipple touches their mouth, but who will begin rooting frantically at the feel of a silicone teat.

So depending on the circumstances, offering supplements by bottle may have an impact on continued breastfeeding. The most obvious way to avert potential problems is to avoid bottles where possible. There are a number of ways of doing this:

- Cup-feeding. Many hospitals now recognise the risk of early bottle introduction, and a cup is often their preferred method of supplementation. A small vessel like a medicine cup with a rim is used to enable the baby to lap the milk. Cup-feeding is most suitable for premature babies and very young newborns who only need a few ml. Term babies instinctively put their hands up to their mouths when hungry and trying to find their food source, so they often end up wriggling about and knocking the cup, spilling valuable expressed milk.

  Another problem with cup feeding is that it requires good tongue movement and co-ordination to lap. Yet a lot of babies need supplementation precisely because they're struggling with this and can't feed effectively at the breast. Parents may then tip the cup to pour milk into the baby's mouth. This can result in coughing, spluttering and potential aspiration if baby doesn't coordinate a swallow with the unexpected influx of milk. This is particularly problematic for a baby receiving a formula supplement, as aspiration could lead to inflammation and potentially infection.

Large volumes can sometimes be quickly swallowed from the cup when it's used to pour milk, and this can also be habit forming.

Many parents report low satisfaction levels from cup-feeding after the first day or two, and find it tricky – particularly in the middle of the night. The risk is that bottles are introduced as a result. Cup feeding is most suitable in a hospital setting, for supplementing premature babies and during the first 48 hours of life when the volumes of milk needed are small.

- Finger-feeding is another option not often discussed by hospitals, but listed as an acceptable method in the NICE guidelines. The caregiver allows baby to suck a clean, upturned finger, while a supplement of milk is delivered into the corner of the mouth via a fine tube or syringe. As the baby is already sucking the finger, any milk introduced to his mouth is automatically swallowed.

Hospitals aren't typically fans of this approach, as multiple people putting fingers in a baby's mouth, and equipment that is more expensive and difficult to clean, increases infection risks. Some health professionals worry that parents will deliver the milk too quickly, or plunge the entire syringe if they cough or sneeze (yes, this was what one couple I worked with were told).

However, if parents finger-feed and wash their hands thoroughly beforehand, there is no evidence of any increase in problems. In my experience parents tend to deliver milk slowly until they become confident, and it can be much easier to give larger amounts than with a cup. Many parents report high satisfaction levels.

- Supplementary nursing system (SNS). This works like finger-feeding, except the tube is used at the breast instead of the finger. You can buy specialist ready-to-use systems that may be more suitable for long-term use or out and about, but many lactation specialists will fashion them from a narrow naso-gastric tube and a bottle. Baby needs to be latching and suckling well enough to pull milk through the system and so it isn't suitable for all.

  Some lactation specialists love the SNS, but like every other method of supplementation they carry risks if used inappropriately. Whereas other supplementation methods don't involve breastfeeding, with an SNS we are potentially changing the mechanics of breastfeeding; some babies can quickly become hooked on the overly fast flow, the feel of the tube in their mouth, the sound of it emptying... and then become fussy when the tube isn't in situ.

  Many claim that an SNS will stimulate mum's breasts and help her supply, but if baby has shallow attachment, and is mainly pulling milk from the tube rather than triggering the milk ejection reflex, then I'm not sure it's effective. Some mums don't express because they believe the stimulation from using the SNS is sufficient, but in my experience it's often not enough to maintain or increase supply if baby isn't feeding effectively.

For parents who want to use bottles, it can be hard to know which to choose. Most bottles claim to be close or closer to a breast, and often for different reasons. A baby that is feeding well should be able to take a standard bottle just as well as any of the fancy models. If you find yourself shopping around for different teats because your baby is struggling, seek some support to assess whether he is using the appropriate mouth and tongue action.

For newborns trying to establish breastfeeding, if a bottle is used I generally find latex teats (if no allergies) make for an easier transition back to the breast. Some silicone teats that are supposedly 'like nipples' are long, hard and have a hole in the end; if the newborn experiences this he may make no connection with the soft, supple feeling of a mother's nipple.

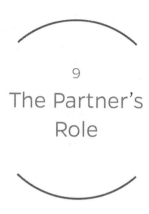

9

The Partner's Role

During antenatal sessions, parents often raise the subject of sharing feeds. Before children both partners often work outside the home, and couples commonly divide chores such as cooking and cleaning between them. It's not uncommon to hear mums saying things along the lines of:

'I want my partner to be able to get involved in the feeding so they can bond.'

'We're going to mix feed so we can both do night feeds.'

'We plan to introduce a bottle ASAP so we're sharing all aspects of caring for baby.'

These statements all sound perfectly logical, don't they? Feeding is bonding, and of course all modern-day parents share day-to-day duties; it's not the 1950s. It isn't equal if one person does all the night feeds while the other sleeps; particularly when mums have carried the baby and given birth. Mums need rest and it's natural that those who care for her want to help. What we need to ask is, 'What is the best way to do this?'

Does feeding promote bonding?

Let's unpick this question of feeding and bonding. I know it's widely accepted that feeding a baby is bonding, but who decided this? Is it because we consider the act of giving food and nourishment nurturing? Do parents actually find bottle-feeding *more* of a bonding experience than other things they could do with their baby? Could it be considered key to bonding just because of the culture we live in?

If we ask expectant parents to describe what they imagine feeding their baby will be like, they generally describe a calming, enjoyable experience. They typically use words that highlight eye contact and touch – connecting, loving behaviours.

Most of the infant feeding we see in society uses formula and bottles. Children play at feeding their dolls, popular TV shows, celebrities, adverts, magazines and news features all present imagery that reinforces the bottle-feeding message. Gradually the concept of bottle feeding being linked with positive emotions has developed.

A 2016 study examining how infant feeding was portrayed in British women's magazines looked at the content of five of the bestselling women's weekly magazines over a four-month period. There was only one visual representation of breastfeeding, compared with 11 of bottle-feeding. The magazines also reported numerous barriers to breastfeeding, including concerns about adverse health consequences. The authors concluded:

> An improvement in visual representations of and factual information about breastfeeding may be helpful in re-defining social norms about infant feeding.

We can add this to what we know about babies and

breastfeeding. As breastfeeding triggers the release of hormones associated with love and connection, it's well documented that breastfeeding is bonding. Given the culture around us, many of us mentally extrapolate this information to assume that feeding a baby is bonding, whether it's by breast or bottle.

Suggesting that a parent must bottle-feed to bond is just as inaccurate as saying a parent must breastfeed to bond. There are plenty of exclusively breastfed babies who are extremely bonded to their non-lactating parent; there are people with disabilities who physically can't breastfeed their babies who are perfectly bonded and there are lots of people who simply choose not to breastfeed who are bonded too.

The real assumption I think we have to question is whether an act that attemps to *mimic* breastfeeding is the most effective way of releasing bonding, relaxing, connecting hormones in partners. As you would expect, much of the research that has been done focuses on dads and male hormones.

Towards the end of their partner's pregnancy, men who are actively involved in fathering often experience a drop in testosterone levels and an increase in prolactin levels. This reduces sex drive and may contribute to a reduction in aggressive or competitive behaviour. Some theorise that historically this would have reduced the chances of the father seeking another mate outside of the family unit.

After birth prolactin levels in fathers spike, which is thought to further promote gentle, family-orientated behaviour. Levels remain significantly elevated throughout the first year, and appear to have the potential to reorganise neurological pathways over time, to encourage continued connection with the family.

Fathers also experience an increase in oxytocin, which can reduce their response to social stress. In animals this hormone is shown to inhibit defensive behaviour and cause them to seek attachment and close proximity to others. One study found that artificial oxytocin caused men to rank their partner as more attractive, but not strangers or colleagues.

So bonding, caring, nurturing behaviours are linked with hormones. The next question has to be: what can influence these hormone levels in partners?

- Oxytocin is produced in both sexes and is initiated in the same way, by holding, touching, kissing and interaction. The more oxytocin is flowing, the more empathic all parties may be (which as any tired, short-tempered parents can confirm, can only help). A 2009 study found that the more dads cuddled their babies, the more their oxytocin levels rose. Researchers described the process as being like a positive feedback loop; the more you touch, the more oxytocin you have; the more oxytocin, the more you touch. There also appears to be a correlation between the oxytocin levels of couples. By studying mum's levels researchers could predict the father's levels later on.

- Vasopressin is another hormone released in response to close contact and touch. It's thought to play a significant role in driving male behaviour. It's nicknamed the 'monogamy hormone' and serves a number of functions; it helps dad to recognise his baby and seek attachment both with his baby and its mother. Fathers who produce higher levels of vasopressin appear more dedicated to their partners and express more protective behaviours, while displaying less anxiety and aggression.

Touch, contact, gazing into baby's eyes, warmth, being

involved and interacting promote bonding, just like in other human relationships. Parents who want exclusively breastfed babies can do all of these things without a bottle.

Good dads do night feeds...

Society is hot on the idea that good partners do night feeds. This message is one that formula companies appear keen to promote, because sharing feeds is really quite difficult if only one person produces milk. Bottles of formula, on the other hand, mean the other person can do 'their share'.

Formula marketing often reaffirms this notion, with images of dad feeding the baby, or 'promising to do his share of night feeds'. It's a successful marketing angle because they're tapping into both of the notions we've discussed: 'good dads' take an active role in the home; and feeding is bonding. The whole concept actually undermines women, but masquerades as feminist 'equality'.

However, is it right to say that 'equal' means splitting every task in half? When I load the dishwasher, should I leave half for my partner to load so it's 'fair', or does it make more sense for me to finish loading and for him to put the clean pots away when it's done? In some families perhaps one person always loads the dishwasher, while the other tackles the laundry. One person might do both those tasks while the other does the ironing and takes out the bins.

Sometimes it makes more sense to share tasks based on strengths. For example, in my house we don't take it in turns fixing a shelf because I live with someone with great woodwork skills. This means he can do a better job in a quarter of the time. I think, without being at all discriminatory, that it's fair to say I'm in a stronger position to breastfeed a baby than my partner is. So is 'sharing the feeding' automatically the best way for everyone to get their needs met?

One mum commented: 'Frankly I think my husband's parenting skills are in no way diminished by his physiological inability to lactate, and find it a bit insulting that he has to be 'included in this way, as if he has no other role.'

How practical is it for a non-lactating parent to share night feeds if baby is exclusively breastfed?

For someone else to do a night feed, a breastfeeding mum would need to express milk in advance. When baby is young, many mums struggle to express enough for a full feed in one expressing session. Pumping is a learnt art that can take time to perfect, and if mum isn't missing a feed but removing extra milk on top, she may need to express multiple times to obtain enough for a whole feed. If mums are expecting to quickly pump enough milk to replace a feed, they may worry they're not producing enough when this doesn't happen.

Many parents don't realise that, even using an extremely effective, high-tech hospital-grade double pump, if mum hasn't been shown effective techniques for expressing she might be removing less than half the milk she actually has available. Other mums can rapidly express larger volumes, but if mum has an ample supply then, rather than missing a feed and sleeping soundly while baby is fed the expressed milk, she may get so full that she ends up needing to express at the same time baby gets a bottle for her own comfort.

If a mum with no feeding or supply problems begins to express before breastfeeding is considered 'established' at around the six-week mark, it can kick-start over-production of milk because her body is being asked for more milk than usual. While this can be handy if it's planned for a return to work, it's not so useful for a new mum wondering why she has enough milk to feed half the babies on her street.

Many mums dislike expressing, some babies hate bottles

and sharing the feeding can end up being a lot more work than mum just breastfeeding the baby and finding another way to maximise her sleep.

The other problem that is often not mentioned is the 'mum radar' or 'mumdar'. When you're a newly lactating mum, your breasts are like a highly tuned sensor on a hair trigger. When baby wants feeding they go into overdrive; mums often report that they wake up with their breasts tingling just before baby stirs. So mum may be disturbed and awake even if someone else is feeding. Add to this the frequency with which small babies often feed and it makes a long unbroken sleep stretch for mum even more tricky, unless you live in a mansion and she can take herself off to a separate wing.

As baby gets older and partners return to work, often it's a lot easier to breastfeed at night than it is for either person to bottle-feed. If baby is in a co-sleeping cot attached to the side of the bed, nobody even has to sit up. Compare this to the requirements for preparing formula milk safely at 3am (see chapter 5).

What about help during the night?
Feeding is just a small part of night-time parenting. Some like to hold baby tummy-to-tummy after the feed, so they can stroke baby's back to give a gentle winding and a few minutes for milk to settle. Newborns fill their nappy often too, so night-time nappies are up for grabs. Partners can also take care of mum, perhaps by fetching a drink or fixing a snack if needed. In the early days mum might need help to get baby in a comfortable position, or to adjust pillows to help her feed in a reclined or side-lying position.

Many parents aren't aware that a couple of studies have shown that exclusive breastfeeding actually *maximises* sleep quality. A study from 2004, looking at sleep duration, found that exclusively breastfeeding mothers slept approximately 20 minutes longer than mothers who were mix feeding. Over 24 hours of day and night, sleep levels among breastfeeding mothers were comparable with mixed-feeding and exclusively formula-feeding mums. Another study found that breastfeeding mothers got an average of 182 minutes of slow-wave sleep, compared to 63 minutes for those exclusively bottle-feeding. Slow-wave sleep is an important marker of sleep quality, and those with a higher percentage of slow-wave sleep report less daytime fatigue.

This can mean that after the early weeks, when partners return to work and might not be able to be quite so hands on during the night (perhaps they have a job that requires them to be on the ball at work), there's less work all round if you're breastfeeding.

However, it's really about finding what works for your family unit. While it's not often talked about, parents of babies past the newborn stage often tell me that mum and baby sleep in one room during the week, while the other parent hits the spare room (or the newly decorated nursery!), returning to the family bed at weekends and taking over more night-time duties. This allows both parents to be better rested and in turn have more time for each other.

For others that wouldn't work, or a different arrangement works better; but slicing baby care straight down the middle is rarely as easy in practice as it might sound in theory.

Ensuring everyone gets enough rest to function is important. Exclusive breastfeeding can make it feel as though a lot of the responsibility sits with mum, but that needn't be so. While the early days when everyone is learning may be difficult, breastfeeding soon becomes second nature for everyone involved. Mums can also maximise their sleep at other times of day:

- The 'keep an eye out'. When mums breastfeed, many experience a surge of the hormone oxytocin which can result in them feeling very sleepy. If help is on hand, this can be the perfect opportunity for mum to rest. If someone can sit close by or cuddle up during the feed to keep an eye on baby so mum doesn't need to, it can allow her to relax, knowing baby is safe even if she falls into a deep sleep. After the feed the helper can either hold baby for some skin-to-skin time while mum sleeps, or ensure both are in a safe sleep space if it's naps all round.
- The dawn shift – AKA collect and deliver. Instead of expressing, some find it works for mum to feed before dad takes baby into another room so she can sleep, delivering baby back when hunger strikes. By the time baby is a few weeks old, mums can often feed without waking fully, especially with assistance. As an added bonus the hormones released during the feed help mum drift back off to sleep. It's particularly common for parents to do this for the dawn waking at weekends to afford mum a longer sleep stretch.

How important is partner support?

Whether mum breastfeeds is heavily linked to the support (or lack of it) she receives from those around her, and in particular those closest to her. Research repeatedly suggests that the maternal social support network is one of the most influential factors.

Establishing breastfeeding can take time, emotions can run high (fuelled by hormones and sleep disturbances), and paternity or partner leave may be woefully short. This can make it seem urgent to get everything resolved before mum is left to 'cope alone'. It can be incredibly stressful for partners to come home from work to find mum distressed, emotionally wrung out, exhausted and the baby fretful.

The problem is that most partners have little idea how to physically help with breastfeeding. It's often barely covered at antenatal classes, and even then the role of support may be underplayed. In this scenario, suggesting formula to 'give mum a break' can seem obvious. Many have no idea what impact this can have in the early weeks, nor do they realise that 'help' in the form of a bottle can compound whatever problem mum was having, not to mention undermining her confidence. In the longer term it can cause far more problems than it appeared to solve.

Many are not aware of the risks of not breastfeeding for baby or mum, or the impact of a bottle of artificial milk. This can put a lot of pressure on a mum who feels torn: she knows breastfeeding is best, but feels she has no option or way to cope. How many couples get good breastfeeding education prior to having a baby?

What can partners do to support breastfeeding, mum and bond with baby?

I'm firmly of the opinion that having a breastfed baby is the responsibility of everyone connected to baby, not just the mum. Here are some pointers for partners or helpers:

- Learn what you can beforehand. It's easy to assume that breastfeeding is easy, because it's what women have been doing for millennia. If you want to breastfeed, you just pick the baby up and go ahead. Right? In some cases of course this is true. However, sometimes it can be really hard initially, just like when we first get behind the wheel of a car; it takes practice and patience before we feel confident on a busy road. Searching online for video clips or practical information from websites, reading books and attending any groups or sessions running locally can be really helpful. One dad I met recently had watched a technical 'how to' video and had mastered hand-expressing far more effectively than mum had. As they needed some extra milk on hand, expressing became his job (while mum ate chocolates and preened baby).

- If mum needs support when baby arrives, go with her. Partners can be invaluable when seeking breastfeeding support, for several reasons. New mums can struggle to retain information; her brain is flooded with bonding, nurturing hormones that prompt care-giving maternal behavior. Some partners are particularly good at visualising angles and remembering tips and tricks. One mum I worked with struggled with the timing of breast compressions, a technique used to help push milk down to baby. She would forget to release her hold, or squeeze the breast when baby sucked. With his hand over hers, her partner would gently remind her to 'squeeze now', or say 'OK, release. She's resting'. This short-term teamwork meant bottles and formula weren't needed in this case. Partners also have a different view from mum, who is looking down on things. In clinic we often ask mum to recreate the feed position and attachment without our help, to ensure she can do it at home. Dads can often be heard giving pointers to help.
- Skin-to-skin. This produces bonding and relaxing hormones so you feel 'loved up'.
- Take a bath or shower. Ditch the baby bath and hop

in together. Warm water and skin contact releases even more oxytocin, and most young babies find a skin-to-skin bath or shower more relaxing than going it alone.

- Wearing baby in a sling or baby carrier. Popping baby in a good baby carrier or sling can give dad some close-contact time with baby and give mum a chance to have a bath and a snooze. Nobody needs to go outdoors; slings can be great for pottering round the house. The well-known carriers sold in high-street shops are not always the most comfortable for the job. What works for you depends on your size, shape, and where you find it most comfortable to have the weight distributed, not to mention what you prefer aesthetically. Many areas now have 'sling libraries', where you can try on and hire different carriers before you splurge, and there are also options for hiring online. Although babies might look small, when you've held one for several hours you develop muscles you didn't know existed! There are some important safety guidelines to follow when you wear your baby in a sling or baby carrier called the 'TICKS rule'. You can find this online or at a sling library.

- Cooking and cleaning. If mum is feeding baby and someone makes food for her, everyone gets to eat. New babies do bring mess and chaos, and dishes can start to pile up as nappies and a pile of muslins takes over. This is all normal and can wait, but some mums find it difficult to relax in an untidy home without the urge to start cleaning. If your partner is like this, telling them to ignore the mess and focus on the baby can be impossible. While it's not an option for all, one mum recently told me she'd cut down the baby

list to bare essentials and requested gift vouchers for
a cleaner to cover a few hours in the week following
the birth of their baby. While some will think this
ridiculous and others unnecessary, this mum had
limited time with her partner at home and didn't want
either of them to have to think about housework for a
few days.

- Massage – mum. An upper back and shoulder
massage before a feed can be excellent in the early
days; often mums hunch their shoulders when trying
to breastfeed, resulting in tension across the shoulders
and the back of the neck. There is also an acupressure
point between the shoulder blades near the neck,
linking the nerves in the upper spine with the breast;
massaging this can help trigger the milk ejection
reflex (letdown). At the very least mum should end
up feeling more relaxed. Reminding mum to lean
back and drop her shoulders when feeding baby can
also help.

- Massage – baby. Baby massage may help to regulate
baby's digestive, respiratory and circulatory systems,
as well as helping to soothe trapped wind. It can also
be a lovely way for a parent to connect with baby.
There are lots of online resources and books available,
and in some areas there are weekly classes.

- Music and movement. A 2010 study found that infants
respond to the rhythm and tempo of music and find
it more engaging than speech. Babies appear to enjoy
moving in time to the music and, according to parents,
sometimes have the most unlikely tastes in music.

- Acting as a protector. For cavewomen this might
have meant protection from a dangerous predator;
nowadays we mean protection from general

interference from a host of well-meaning people. If mum's partner is her champion, encouraging and helping her if problems arise, she's far more likely to meet her breastfeeding goals.

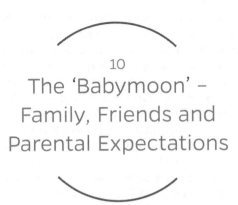

10
The 'Babymoon' – Family, Friends and Parental Expectations

While the trend in recent years has been to celebrate mothers getting back into their skinny jeans as soon as possible, perfectly presented and generally not looking as though they have just spent nine months growing another human, things are shifting. More and more couples are reclaiming the time often referred to as the 'babymoon'. This is a period after the birth when the parents can bond with their baby and be looked after by those around them. It is common in many cultures in some form or another. The aim is that the new mum rests, eats well and only has to focus on mothering her newborn.

Historically, the period of rest after birth has become progressively shorter. Hundreds of years ago it was considered normal for women to stay in bed for three or four weeks, which was called the 'lying in' period. Many in the UK today can remember when women remained in hospital for a couple of weeks after delivery. While new mothers are not usually ill, and do not need to be bed-bound in hospital, I do think that western women get a raw deal when it comes to the postpartum period.

Last year I visited a family and consulted the mother in her bedroom. Various female relatives attended her throughout. She was given a foot massage, food and snacks appeared regularly, someone passed her a burp cloth when needed and another brushed her hair. She was treated like a goddess as a stream of visitors celebrated and ate and drank downstairs. Mum explained that this was common in the Pakistani community, and while there was always a houseful of people, it was extremely rare for the mother and her baby to be disturbed or separated.

This struck me as a contrast to our culture, where often the expectant mum is the focus until baby arrives, at which point the focus shifts to the baby and whether they're thriving, settled and happy. But if we mother the mother, she can better nurture her baby. Home-cooked foods, in comparison to the sandwiches and ready meals tired new parents may depend on, can supply vitamins and minerals that women need as they rest and recover from the birth.

Thinking and planning for a babymoon in advance can be valuable in prompting expectant parents to consider what will happen once the baby arrives. Often there is so much focus on preparing for the birth that the reality of life with a new baby is hardly thought of.

Some parents find themselves dealing with a constant stream of visitors arriving for cuddles with the new baby, and this can be unexpected and exhausting. Sometimes parents realise later that they would rather have chosen to spend this incredibly special time differently, but got swept along.

Spending time at home as a new family can also make establishing breastfeeding easier. Many mums feel self-conscious feeding in front of certain visitors, and they may try to delay feeds or be particularly discreet, when actually time spent on the sofa, skin-to-skin, would have helped them get breastfeeding established. Being in close contact with her baby allows mum to learn and recognise the first cues that her baby is hungry. For newborns this means starting to stir, opening and closing their mouth, and bringing their hand up to suck their finger or hand. This is the 'get ready to feed me' sign.

Next the baby opens their eyes and starts turning their head with their mouth open, in search of food. This is the ideal time to latch baby to the breast or bottle. A newborn baby held skin-to-skin will start moving towards the breast to attach. If this sign is missed, baby will progress to squirming, fussing and eventually crying. For newborns, crying can cause them to be 'disorganised'. This is a frantic state in which they find it much harder to attach and feed well, and they may need calming before they can latch.

If baby is spending lots of time with relatives, it can be harder for mum to spot and respond to these early signs. Some mums say they feel awkward asking for their baby back when well-meaning relatives try to soothe them.

There are many different ways to babymoon, depending on your wants and needs, family situation and the support you have. Below are some ideas: some will likely appeal, while others won't be for you. It's perfectly possible for friends and relatives to be supportive and involved, and protect breastfeeding too.

- Some families choose to set a period of time to spend alone before any non-essential visits (e.g. those that aren't healthcare professionals). This can vary from a day or two to several days or longer.
- Some families choose to set a period of time for only 'VIP' relatives to be around, such as parents and grandparents, or maybe really close friends, who will help cook, tidy and care for the parents, before they

invite anyone else.

- Some families pin a note to the front door asking not to be disturbed unless it's for a delivery. Or they put a note up when mum and baby are sleeping, to deter neighbours or casual visitors if it's inconvenient.

- Some parents find inviting relatives for longer stretches of several hours can be easier overall than flying visits. People can often arrange to just 'pop in', conscious that mum needs to rest, but numerous people doing so can mean a steady stream of short visits. It can be harder for parents to feel they can decline to offer a cuddle with baby if they know the visitor is leaving soon, which can make it tricky if they arrive right before a feed. If they're there for a while they can hold baby after a feed when he's full, relaxed and mum isn't at risk of missing cues.

- In contrast, some parents find longer visits exhausting, and much prefer clarifying in advance that shorter visits are OK but lengthy stays are not. All families are different and it's about each family deciding what works for them.

- Consider accepting any offers of food. Very often family and friends offer help, but we're too polite to accept, or we give them the nice job of holding the baby while we tackle the dishes or the vacuuming. I met a lovely family recently who asked their friends to gift a meal instead of buying things for the baby. Every day a home-cooked dish was left on their doorstep with just a knock to say it was ready. The family planned to host a gathering to cook for their friends and introduce them to the baby when they felt ready. If something like this doesn't appeal or isn't feasible, another option might be to bulk-cook family meals during pregnancy and freeze extras ready for later.

- Parents of older children may arrange for help with school runs, and prepare as much in advance as possible so they don't need to give it brain space post-baby. I knew one mum who picked out in advance seven outfits for the week that followed (based on what activities happened on each day), including socks and underwear. She popped them in ziplock bags with the days of the week written on the front and added anything else needed for that day (like ballet shoes) so that they could literally grab the bags and go.

It's really all about trying to plan in advance to make time to relax, heal and gradually transition to life as a new family unit.

Parental expectations

Impending parenthood provokes a different response in each of us, and often a combination of emotions. Excitement and happiness at the impending arrival can be mixed with uncertainty and even panic. Our expectations of what's to come and what is 'best' and 'normal' are naturally based on what we experience around us. For many of us, smaller families may mean fewer memories of siblings as young babies to draw upon. Even those with lots of experience caring for young babies can find that having their own baby presents unexpected challenges. So we look to those closest to us, or turn to books, magazines, websites and health professionals for advice, all of whom have different opinions, but who nonetheless may plant seeds of expectation in our minds.

Before baby arrives it's common for parents to believe that their baby will be the happiest baby around. As long as you change their nappy when it's soiled, feed them when they're hungry and provide a nice cot and nursery for sleep, your baby won't need to cry because their needs will be met. And for some this may be true.

The reality, however, is that this isn't how parenting a newborn looks for many, many parents, particularly in the early months. Those parents will testify that being the parent of a newborn baby can be incredibly hard.

Even after running through the list of 'needs' and checking all are met, your baby may still cry. The comfy bed you lovingly prepared might as well be covered in nine-inch nails, as they flail and wail every time you try and gently lower them in. Instead of being snuggled on the sofa, you are taking it in turns to pace and jiggle a squirmy, windy baby, before one of you tries to eat one-handed so that the other can have a powernap before shift change.

And the nights – who knew they could be so long? Even when you have everything 'perfect', still baby wriggles, grunts and wants to feed *again*; how can this be when it was only two hours since we just did all this?

I don't feel that long spells of crying should be just accepted as 'colic'; it's always worth seeking help to explore why baby is crying if you're concerned. Sometimes baby is sucking in extra air when they're feeding, or is drinking more lactose (sugar) rich milk because their latch isn't quite deep enough, meaning a small tweak can make a huge difference.

Looking at your expectations can be really important. Are they realistic? If not, adapting them can be a whole lot easier than trying to change a normal newborn. Furthermore, given that parents have the cognitive ability to adapt, rather than the immature neurological pathways a baby has, it would also seem to be the fairer option. Expectations can play a big part in how parents perceive their baby's behaviour.

Newborn norms:

- Feeding and waking frequently day and night.
  Babies have no concept of time, and take time to
  adjust to feeding at spaced intervals rather than
  continuously via the placenta. Breastmilk changes
  composition at night to include more of the
  hormones that induce sleep, and helps baby develop
  circadian rhythms (sleep patterns).

  If parents know to expect frequent feeding at night,
  they can better prepare for it. Some choose to use a cot
  attached to the bed so nobody has to sit up, get up or
  try and keep themselves awake. Instead they can slide
  baby over then feed lying down. This can also help
  prevent triggering baby's startle reflex, which kicks in
  when they're lowered down (and think they're falling),
  and with practice sometimes this can be done with
  everyone barely rousing.

- Evening cluster feeding. It's common for babies of
  a few weeks old to want frequent or constant feeds,
  usually in the early to mid-evening, after which baby
  takes a longer sleep stretch. In babies, suckling releases
  a hormone called cholecystokinin (CCK), and after a
  feed they have high levels of CCK. This makes them
  feel relaxed and sated, but as levels drop again 10 to
  20 minutes later, baby may signal to feed again. Babies
  appear to go through this loop a number of times
  before settling into a deeper sleep. As breastmilk is
  typically digested within 2–3 hours, some experts
  theorise that cluster feeding is needed so that baby can
  pack lots of breastmilk into their digestive system to
  sustain the longer sleep that follows.

  Knowing cluster feeding is normal can allow some
  planning. This might involve a second parent hopping

in the bath with the baby, or wearing a carrier for some skin-to-skin time with baby earlier in the evening, while mum builds a nest of pillows, snacks, books, drinks, music/TV remote… ready to settle down for a longer feeding session later.

In contrast, if parents are expecting to feed their newborn, then put them down for a few hours while they eat and have some time 'hands free', and they haven't been told about cluster feeding, they may believe there is a problem and baby is not getting enough to eat.

- Need for contact: newborns expect contact as they transition from life in the womb, with constant movement, water-muffled sounds and security, to the outside world. Familiar voices, smells and touch can help ease baby through the transition period many now refer to as the fourth trimester.

At times it's hard to pick apart instinct and social expectations. It's always worth remembering that a baby simply doesn't have sufficient neurological pathways to attempt to manipulate or control – they're working much more instinctively. Ample evidence shows that meeting the needs of an infant leads to long-term security, compared to the potentially negative implications of trying to train a baby's behaviour to suit the parents. Babies don't develop mature sleep rhythms until they're several months old, so they're not developing 'habits' at the newborn stage, they're purely focused on survival.

Even with the most realistic expectations, some babies will still be much more intense than others, and their parents can still be exhausted and overwhelmed.

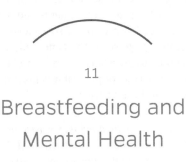

11

Breastfeeding and Mental Health

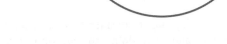

The relationship between infant feeding and mental health is incredibly complex, not least because pregnancy, birth and other factors that can result in stress, trauma or post-traumatic stress can influence how mum feels before she starts breastfeeding. Add to this any pre-existing mental health history and it becomes much more difficult to tease apart cause and correlation.

It's common for mums to say that they felt their mental health improved once they stopped breastfeeding. Some say that we should stop talking to mums about the reasons for breastfeeding, because this puts pressure on them – which isn't good for their mental health. As I hope I've demonstrated so far in this book, it's really not quite that simple.

What's interesting is that evidence consistently suggests that not breastfeeding can significantly increase the risk of postnatal depression (PND), particularly if mum wanted and intended to breastfeed. A 2014 study of over 10,000 mums found that those who didn't plan to breastfeed and indeed gave formula from birth (let's call them group 1) were overall significantly more likely to become depressed than those who planned to breastfeed and who did so exclusively for at least four weeks (group 2). However, the same study also found that those who planned to breastfeed yet failed to do so (group 3), were at even higher risks of postnatal depression than group 1. As a result the authors stressed:

> the importance of both providing expert breastfeeding support to women who want to breastfeed; but also, of providing compassionate support for women who had intended to breastfeed, but who find themselves unable to.

One group that this study didn't consider was those who planned to breastfeed, and were doing so, but who were also experiencing severe problems. We need to explore the emotional impact of this situation too, so that we can identify the difference between those feeling vulnerable because they're experiencing a stressful or distressing situation they don't know how to resolve, and those who have PND.

A lack of support when mums have problems can be very frustrating. One mum described it:

> I was so angry. I put my cards on the table with the GP and told him how desperate I was to breastfeed. I explained how frustrated I was that nobody seemed able to help me stop the pain; that I had been treated for mastitis and thrush (now several times), but still it hurt. I told him repeatedly that no, I didn't think it would be better all-round to just 'give a bottle'.
>
> He replied by asking me if I thought I might have PND! I was so pissed off at this point that I promptly burst into tears, probably convincing him further that I

had the 'baby blues'. But I was just so frustrated that yet again I wasn't going to get help with actually solving the problem and he was so bloody patronising, that's why I was crying.

If someone is living in a stressful situation day after day, week after week, can we really expect them to be happy? I want to stress that there are some wonderful, sensitive, kind doctors out there, I'm not suggesting all are so dismissive; yet we also have to recognise this is what some mothers experience.

How are breastfeeding and PND linked?
The mechanism that potentially connects not breastfeeding and PND is not yet understood, but there are several proposed theories:

1. When a baby is breastfeeding effectively, mum has hormonal surges of both oxytocin and prolactin. These hormones can help her to feel more relaxed, less anxious and at times (particularly in the early days) very sleepy. Prolactin levels remain elevated when breastfeeding, reducing gradually as baby weans.
2. Depression has been associated with inflammation, and breastfeeding helps to modulate the body's inflammatory response. The 2007 study that put forward this theory also noted that: 'Breastfeeding difficulties such as nipple pain can increase the risk of depression and must be addressed promptly.' The inflammatory response theory is also interesting if we consider what happens when milk transfer from mum to baby isn't as effective as it could be. A mum with an abundant milk supply may find herself with lumpy breasts, blockages and a persistent low level

of inflammation. When this happens mums report feeling run-down, tired and emotional – issues that often resolve as soon as their breasts are drained.

3. The most controversial theory to date is one that was published in 2009 by a team of psychologists in a journal called *Medical Hypotheses and Ideas*. The authors outline a theory in the context of an emerging discipline known as 'evolutionary medicine', proposing that not breastfeeding 'unwittingly mimics conditions associated with the death of an infant'. They suggest that biologically the only time a mammal wouldn't lactate would be in the case of infant loss, a well-documented trigger for depression. They note the evidence suggests that bottle-feeding mothers hold their babies more than their breastfeeding peers – as is seen in bereaved mammals. Critics of this theory (of which there are many) point out that non-breastfeeding mums may simply hold their babies more to increase bonding and attachment. The touch and contact may be to help release the nurturing hormones normally experienced when breastfeeding.

When we consider all the above in combination with the lack of effective support some mums receive, we have an even bigger problem. When mums tell me their breastfeeding stories, it's extremely common to hear that they 'feel like they're going mad'. What they often mean is that their gut feeling is that something isn't quite right with the feeding (be that breast or bottle), but everyone around her is adamant that it's fine.

Sometimes mum can be certain that things aren't fine, for example if she has nipple damage or pain. Similarly, a bottle-feeding mum may see milk spilling from the corners of her baby's mouth, and note that other people's babies don't do the same. But at other times feeding problems are much more subtle; perhaps her baby is happy during the day, yet seems to be in discomfort and squirms or cries for long periods at night. Perhaps she feels he isn't taking as much milk as he could; falling asleep quickly yet rousing as soon as he's unlatched. Other times it's just a feeling she has.

We should listen more carefully to mothers. They know far more than many (including themselves) give them credit for, because their instincts, combined with the fact they are with their baby much more than anyone helping them, mean they have an invaluable insight others don't. Mums, however, often report feeling concerned that their healthcare providers consider them neurotic or anxious; that they will be dismissed as a first-time mum or, if they've had other children, that people will think she should know what she's doing.

I think the problem here is that mothers are seeing medical healthcare professionals, when often there is nothing significantly medically wrong with the baby. The medics see a thriving, healthy baby, who is often smiley and distracted when out and about; these babies aren't 'ill' in a medical sense. They don't see the baby who screamed hourly while writhing around struggling to take a feed the previous night. Mums often bring mobile phone footage as evidence, but still struggle to get their concerns taken seriously. If they do, despite NICE guidance stating the first 'intervention' should be for someone appropriately qualified to fully assess a feed, a recent poll I ran on Facebook suggested this rarely happens. Instead the medical model turns to medications and hypoallergenic formulas, which at times are essential, but often parents report minimal or no real difference at all once they are introduced, and there can be knock-on effects for breastfeeding.

Unfortunately, sometimes women feel dismissed as emotional, distressed or tired when they seek support for a baby doctors don't perceive to be unwell. Some say their concerns were taken more seriously when dad took baby to the appointment or attended with them. It is clear that very few new mums feel truly empowered – regardless of how they feed their baby.

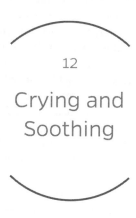

12

Crying and Soothing

Crying babies are an interesting subject and it's fascinating to watch how different parents react to a red-faced, flailing, wailing bundle. Crying is just one of a few communication tools at a young baby's disposal.

We hear a lot about the different cries babies have, and how the art is in identifying which cry means what so you can respond accordingly. There are now devices and apps that claim to help 'decode' infant cries, with the rationale that if the cry isn't a 'hungry cry', the baby doesn't need the breast (again making the incorrect assumption that the breast is just food).

It's true that some cries are low-pitched, rhythmic and preceded by clear sounds that change depending on the need. Other cries are high-pitched, urgent and tend to make mothers feel a need to deal with their baby quickly – an instinct I believe is there for a reason. It's also true that given time you do instinctively learn to recognise a tired cry from a windy cry, but what I disagree with is the idea that for a breastfeeding mum, it's imperative (in that hazy postpartum fuzz) to have nailed every cry and know the perfect solution ASAP.

I can still clearly remember hovering over my daughter's crib, not rushing to pick her up and trying to listen to the cry to work it out. She (probably confused as to why I was staring at her without actually doing anything), started to turn red in the face and went up a gear in volume. At this point I admitted defeat, offered her the breast and sat down to reread the 'cry descriptions'. Had it been a 'nah, nah', 'wah wah', or 'nah, wah nah'?

For some babies the breast isn't a fix-all, but for many the fact that it meets so many needs can give parents time to naturally get to know their baby and understand their communications better. What's also interesting is that the same cry can provoke a wide range of emotional responses in different mothers. A study exploring how a group of mothers responded to clips of babies crying found that some had visibly increased stress levels, while others didn't. The same recorded cry was perceived by some mothers to be a 'nuisance cry' or one designed to 'manipulate', while other mothers felt it was because the baby needed care. In practice researchers found that those who felt it was a nuisance cry were less responsive to their own infants.

Responsiveness is important for the infant to develop what is called 'secure attachment', which is different to bonding. As the Institute of Health Visiting explains, it is 'the enduring 'tie of affection that the baby develops towards their main carers, usually their parents'. They continue:

> *Infants develop emotional health and wellbeing when they experience loving, sensitive care from their parents or main carers. Securely attached infants have pleasurable interactions with their main carers and can expect comfort when they are distressed.*
>
> *Secure attachment is one of the main sources of later resilience in childhood: infants who are securely*

attached feel safe to play and learn. Securely attached children achieve better outcomes across all domains including social and emotional development, behaviour, relationships with peers, and learning.

How is this relevant to breastfeeding?

A small study in 2011 examined how breastfeeding impacted on mum's responsiveness to her baby two to four weeks postpartum. Mothers were given MRI brain scans, while listening to recordings of their own and other babies crying. Mothers who weren't breastfeeding showed reduced activity in several brain regions, including those the study authors linked with empathy. They also noted that other animal studies have identified links between these brain regions and parenting behaviour.

This is interesting if we consider that formula-fed infants are often perceived to be more settled, contented or less demanding than their breastfed peers. They may sleep more deeply and be considered 'easier' because their patterns (given their static food source), may be much more predictable. However, if we consider that crying is communication, is this 'settled' behaviour normal for a human infant?

A 2012 study explored infant crying in depth. The authors commented:

Humans often perceive infant crying as stress, but for infant animals irritability is a normal component of signalling to parents. The expression of offspring demand is part of a dynamic signalling system between parents and offspring, and has received much attention from zoologists studying a variety of bird and mammal species.

Dr Philip Zeskind, an associate professor of psychology who

has also completed research in this area, agrees:

> *Although breast-fed babies are perceived to be more irritable than bottle-fed newborns, our results suggest that the behaviours of breast-fed infants are physiologically more desirable.*

Why some human babies signal more than others is still up for debate. Some theorise that healthier babies are likely to be more demanding, which helps them maintain proximity to, and elicit care from their parents (smart move if you're a vulnerable newborn), optimising development.

Sometimes babies simply communicate more because they have more to tell us. A newborn who has had an assisted birth with forceps has no way of expressing that she's stiff or sore. Whereas you or I might grab an extra pillow, or turn over to adjust our position, babies can't do this and they have particularly heavy heads in relation to the rest of their body.

Some babies are more sensitive (just like some adults) and take longer to transition to life outside the womb; being the wrong temperature or having a soiled nappy can all be a bit too much. Ultimately what it's important to understand is that babies simply don't have the neurological connections to be capable of manipulation.

Deny the super power of your breasts!

What to do when baby cries is again influenced by living in a non-breastfeeding culture. As we've established, mum's breasts can be food, pacifier and comfort blanket all rolled into one – the ultimate security. Yet society seems scared of this fix-all, and mothers are frequently warned against using this magic tool as part of their parenting arsenal.

'I've heard not to let my baby use me as a dummy or he

will never learn to sleep', has to be one of the phrases most often uttered by parents. The fear that a baby may continue to need them at night, or worse, manipulate their parents into all-night cot parties, terrifies many.

While society is generally fine with a baby being reliant on a pacifier (aka a silicone replica of a nipple), or a comfort blanket or toy, attachment to mum is a different ball game. High-street chemist Boots published a 'Napping dos and don'ts':

> *It's natural for babies to fall asleep after a feed. Nursing or bottle-feeding newborns to sleep is a great bonding experience, but over time it can become the only way they can fall asleep. Try to separate nursing from naps even by just a few minutes; read a story or change baby's nappy in between.*

That's right, Boots – it is natural and bonding, and it releases hormones many struggle to fight. There's no evidence supporting the theory that this becomes 'the only way they can fall asleep'.

Does the idea that if we do what comes naturally, our babies will never be able to fall asleep without feeding really make any sense at all? Before there were such warning leaflets telling parents to 'separate nursing from sleep', did the human race suffer severe sleep problems? What about cultures that aren't given this guidance? Do they have generation upon generation of adults unable to sleep without a breast or bottle? Of course not.

Parents are often bombarded with the message that holding, feeding or comforting their baby at night will lead to some sort of 'bad sleep habit'. They begin to believe this is an established fact, rather than just a well-marketed opinion – usually that of someone charging you money to help train your baby to change his expectations to meet yours, or selling you a product designed to help induce hands-free sleep, such as a vibrating bouncy chair or a rocking stand for a Moses basket.

Where is the evidence that young infants should be able to self-soothe? Who assumed that an infant, completely reliant upon us for everything else, has the skills to put himself to sleep? How do parents decide if and when these skills have developed? Or are we assuming that babies are born with this skill because their sleep is so different in the early months and some infants *appear* to self-soothe then?

What does the science suggest?

A study focusing on self-soothing found there was very little data exploring the development of this skill during the first year of life. So the researchers decided to study infants in four age groups (3, 6, 9, and 12 months) for four nights by using videosomnography (which uses both electrical patterns in the brain and video footage together) to code 'night-time awakenings and parent-child interactions'. They found:

> *A large degree of variability was observed in parents' putting the infant to bed awake or asleep and in responding to vocalizations after nighttime awakenings. Most infants woke during the night at all ages observed. Younger infants tended to require parental intervention at night to return to sleep, whereas older infants exhibited a greater proportion of self-soothing after nighttime awakenings. However, even in the 12-month-old group, 50% of infants typically required parental intervention to get back to sleep after waking. Results emphasize the individual and contextual factors that affect the development of self-soothing behavior during the first year of life.*

In short – parents put their children to bed in different ways; some were responsive to wakenings while others weren't, yet most infants woke at all ages. While more older infants 'self-soothed' than younger ones, even at a year and a half the infants needed help to go back to sleep.

Most sleep literature seems to assume that babies don't want to sleep, and that we have to teach them who is boss otherwise they will be up all night. What is this assumption based on? What if human infants, just like all other mammals, naturally want to sleep, but at times – perhaps when teething or having a developmental burst, or when separated from mum – find it difficult?

What if instead of 'waking for the breast', they actually just wake anyway, and it turns out that the breast is the perfect soothing tool? What if, instead of them fighting sleep, for some reason or other sleep is fighting them?

Concern about 'spoiling babies' can lead to an increased risk of perceiving communications as manipulative and as a result not responding rapidly when baby signals, instead believing baby 'has to learn that sometimes we need to wait'. This stems from something known as behavioural theory or conditioning, which states (in very basic terms) that our actions are driven by the response previously received. If something is rewarded with a nice response, we do it again – and similarly an unpleasant response deters repetition.

This was certainly a popular belief of parenting experts in the early 20th century, upon which many current practices are based. However Dr Eleanor Maccoby and others have since shown that when it comes to babies the theory doesn't hold water.

Another study from Manchester also explored infant crying, and checked in with a group of babies at four periods during the first year of life. The researchers concluded that rapid parental response to crying was associated with significantly less crying overall.

Another consequence of our norm being to feed babies a static, unchanging product, in contrast to the ever-changing make-up of breastmilk – is that their demands are much more predictable. I say 'consequence' as for the breastfeeding dyad expecting consistent patterns is unrealistic. Even if breastmilk was just food, and babies only breastfed for nutrition, they're still consuming a dynamic product that is changing constantly, over periods as short as a single breastfeed, and as long as the entire period of lactation. It's clearly a very different scenario.

We now know that breastmilk composition changes in response to milk removal that occurs during breastfeeding – as in the amount baby transfers at each feed. This means that when formula feeding it can sometimes be easier to predict a feeding pattern, or encourage particular timings in young infants by changing the amount given. In contrast a breastfed baby's pattern may be to feed after 1½ hours, then 3 hours, then 3 hours, then 1 hour, then a few feeds back to back, then 6 hours, and so on.

A 2012 study noted that while many popular childcare books recommend feeding babies to a timed routine, no large-scale study had ever examined the effects of this. After controlling for a wide range of confounders, the authors concluded that babies fed to a schedule, rather than when they signalled, performed around 17 per cent of a standard deviation below demand-fed babies in tests at all ages, and scored four points lower in IQ tests at age eight.

As a result, following baby's lead and feeding on cue is now widely recommended for both breast and bottle-fed babies, and this is included in the new Unicef Baby Friendly Initiative that many health services in the UK adhere to or are working to implement.

Something else that the same study noticed was that mothers who were schedule feeding noted increased levels of maternal wellbeing – which is what many 'experts' use to justify the methods they are suggesting to parents. It's summed up by the oft-quoted phrase 'a happy mum makes a happy baby'.

I don't think it's that simple.

Parenting literature often sells parents the notion that you can have the 'perfect baby' if only you implement the right schedule and parenting techniques. 'Perfect' in this context is of course a predictable, calm baby, who sleeps long stretches by several months of age at the latest.

Mums who have a baby who doesn't conform, perhaps waking and feeding at night longer than one book or another suggests they should, or signaling for a feed every two hours rather than four, therefore report feeling as if they're doing something wrong. They sometimes express frustration that despite being fed, winded and warm, baby still wakes several times per night. Therefore, when baby does begin to behave more in line with their expectations, I would expect some mothers to report an increased sense of wellbeing.

However, I suspect parents are not always aware that science suggests genes may also influence night sleep. A 2013 study of 995 twins at 6, 18, 30 and 48 months of age found that while day sleep could to some degree be influenced by environmental factors, 'Strong genetic influences were found for consolidated nighttime sleep duration.'

Other studies have found that it's perfectly normal for baby to rouse regularly, including one that found babies aged between 2–9 months averaged three major awakenings each night. So how did someone decide babies should or could sleep all night by 4–6 months without signalling to their caregiver?

The reality is that *all* babies, just like other mammals, will transition to independence without being pushed or forced – because it's a natural progression that develops as they mature. The expectations many have of infant sleep can be unrealistic, and are not beneficial from an infant's perspective.

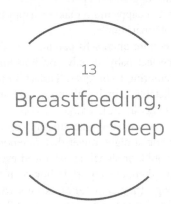

13

Breastfeeding, SIDS and Sleep

Sudden Infant Death Syndrome (SIDS) is the sudden and unexplained death of an infant, where no cause is found after a detailed post mortem. Research into SIDS has been well funded, and as a result safety recommendations have helped to almost halve cases since the 1990s. That said, as it's still the most common cause of death in young infants, it's naturally of concern to parents.

Much SIDS prevention focuses on positioning and safety during sleep; placing baby feet at the foot of the cot, ensuring blankets are ventilated, there are no soft toys, bumpers or pillows and maintaining an appropriate ambient temperature.

While this is all incredibly important, many are surprised to hear that there is any connection between SIDS and feeding method, or presume that it must be insignificant or it would feature in other literature and antenatal classes. In fact, feeding method is so important in terms of the risks of SIDS that the Foundation for the Study of Infant Death (FSID), the UK's leading baby charity working to prevent sudden infant deaths, carries this statement on their website:

> *Research shows that babies who were at least partly breastfed were one-third less likely to die as a cot death than babies who were never breastfed. There are so many reasons why breast is best, but there are none that can be stronger than potentially saving your child's life. We encourage every new mum to breastfeed.*

I decided to dig through the research to see what they had found so compelling. A paper in which researchers analysed the combined result of 23 SIDS studies found that 19 of them linked not breastfeeding to an increased risk of SIDS. Their results also indicated that artificially-fed infants were twice as likely to die as their breastfed peers. A later German study found that not breastfeeding at one month was associated with double the rate of SIDS, with mixed feeding also resulting in an increased risk compared to exclusive breastfeeding. In 2011 another team of researchers combined data from 18 studies and found that the rate of SIDS was 60 per cent lower among infants who had any amount of breastfeeding, compared to those who were fully formula fed. The risk of SIDS was more than 70 per cent lower in infants who had been breastfed exclusively, without any formula, for any period of time.

How not breastfeeding increases SIDS risk is something scientists are still working to establish, but a leading hypothesis is that many cases of SIDS result from defects in protective responses controlled by the brainstem. When everything is working as it should, any 'stressors' to the baby's ability to maintain a constant internal environment trigger his body to respond. The room becoming too warm, for example, would be considered a stressor, because the baby's body needs to work to keep his temperature within a safe range.

Central to this process is a brain chemical called serotonin, which conveys messages between cells and plays a vital role in regulating breathing, heart rate and sleep. One theory which is gathering support is that SIDS victims may be suffering serotonin deficiency, preventing this normal arousal process from taking place. A 2010 study funded by the National Institutes of Health confirmed that SIDS infants did consistently present with abnormally low levels of serotonin and serotonin receptors in the brainstem.

Subsequent investigations demonstrated that babies who died of asphyxia also have deficits in the brain stem serotonin system, and so Professor James Leiter, from the Geisel School of Medicine at Dartmouth, conducted a further study to further explore the serotonin theory. Published in April 2016, it aimed to establish whether exposure to serotonin could shorten apnoea (temporary cessation of breathing), and whether blocking serotonin receptors could have the opposite effect and increase apnoea. In rodents they discovered that exposure could shorten apnoea, but only when a specific type of serotonin receptor was activated – and so the team are now working to ascertain whether this receptor was altered in SIDS victims. Professor Leiter commented:

> Serotonin is important in arousing infants and restoring regular breathing to end apnoeic events when regular breathing is interrupted. Apnoeic events are common in babies, even in healthy babies. Babies seem to be more susceptible to reflexes that suppress breathing, and they need internal processes that stop these apnoeas and restore normal breathing.

Discussion around this theory also ties in with other

techniques shown to be effective in helping to reduce SIDS rates, for example back sleeping and keeping the room at a consistent moderate temperature. If serotonin deficiency results in reduced ability to deal with sleep stressors, reducing sleep stressors should indeed reduce SIDS rates too.

How could feeding method influence serotonin levels?

An amino acid called tryptophan (which is also an antioxidant) is needed to produce serotonin. Colostrum contains 2–3 times more tryptophan than breastmilk and this initial 'loading dose' is thought to be extremely important for appropriate nervous system development.

Tryptophan levels in breastmilk are around double those found in cow's milk and the ratio of tryptophan to other amino acids is also different. This balance of amino acids is key to the way tryptophan is used to make serotonin, which can pass through the blood-brain barrier to be effectively absorbed and utilised.

We know that tryptophan levels in breastmilk aren't static, but are constantly changing throughout the day and for the duration of lactation – as are all the other amino acids. This poses a number of problems for formula manufacturers.

The first is that formula doesn't and can't change; manufacturers must pick a level of tryptophan and stick with it. They can't deliver a higher dose of one ingredient soon after birth and then have it reduce over the coming months, as parents would need a different formula every day.

The second problem is that human milk and cow's milk proteins are really quite different. Human milk is high in a tryptophan-rich protein called α-lactalbumin, which makes up 30 per cent of the total protein content; in contrast, α-lactalbumin makes up around 3 per cent of the protein in cow's milk. In order to provide adequate levels of tryptophan in formula, you have to add more protein. This is why, historically, formula contains significantly higher levels of protein than breastmilk, and is one of the reasons why formula-fed infants typically feed less frequently.

The problem with increasing protein levels in formula is that while it does indeed deliver more tryptophan, it also delivers larger amounts of the other amino acids – resulting in a very different balance than is found in breastmilk. In the infant formula world this is considered a pretty big problem. A paper entitled 'The significance of tryptophan in infant nutrition' states:

> *In the newborn, tryptophan (Trp) and its metabolites are essential to brain maturation and to the development of neurobehavioral regulations of food intake, satiation and sleep-wake-rhythm.*

Not surprisingly, studies have also explored tryptophan levels in formula-fed and breastfed babies. One such paper, which analysed the existing studies, concluded:

> *Current formulas may compositionally meet all requirements, but infants fed those formulas still had plasma amino acid profiles that differed from those in breastfed infants. Plasma concentrations of tryptophan were significantly lower in formula-fed than in breastfed infants in some studies.*

Some manufacturers have been working to add α-lactalbumin to their formula milk. Preliminary research (although some is industry funded) suggests that these experimental formulas may result in increased serotonin production for formula-fed infants, alongside more normal weight gain patterns due to the more normal protein levels. One UK manufacturer started adding α-lactalbumin to infant formula. However, it was removed again when the brand changed hands. I decided to check out the difference in the tryptophan levels in the old formula and new. The formula containing α-lactalbumin lists tryptophan levels at 30mg per 100ml, compared to 23mg per 100ml in the new formulation. (If you're wondering how this sort of adjustment to formula can go on without conclusive research into the health outcomes for babies, read on.)

Of course SIDS risks may yet prove to be unrelated to tryptophan or even serotonin, as the research is ongoing. What is obvious, though, is that formula isn't close to breastmilk, despite the claims of the manufacturers and many parents and healthcare professionals. When formula is thought to be 'closer to breastmilk', which version do we mean? Is it last year's, or the new and improved version? Both are advertised in the same way. Justus von Liebig made the first infant formula in the 1860s:

> *The product consisted of wheat flour, some cow's milk, and malt flour with a little bicarbonate of potash to reduce the acidity of the flours. As a result of his chemical and physiological studies, Liebig determined that these ingredients provided the infant with all the nutritive elements of human milk.*

Formula is ever-evolving, as manufacturers try to replicate and reproduce more and more of the hundreds of constituents breastmilk contains. While it may be closer than it was five, ten or fifteen years ago, the formula of the future will look nothing like that of today.

Waking and sleep training

Most infants who wake up and communicate with their caregivers at night are healthy, put on weight and grow normally; this works well, as a lot of mums need at least one night feed in the early months to maintain a good milk supply. If babies are vulnerable – perhaps their intake is a little low, or if they're premature or very small at term – they may fail to rouse adequately, requiring parents to initiate feeding.

Normal night-time communication, known as 'signalling', is important when talking about infant sleep. The phrase 'sleeping through the night' is actually misleading, as studies using infra-red video recording have shown that infants continue to wake in the night, even if they don't wake their parents. A more accurate phrase would be 'not signalling through the night'. We also have to define what we mean in terms of duration; many books and papers refer to 'sleeping through the night' as 5–6 hours, while others take it to mean 12 hours.

We also need to understand that sleep is not static. Babies may have periods of sleeping longer spells than expected and others of waking more than we might like – it's a common misconception that once baby *can* sleep through the night, they consistently will or should.

Babies are born signalling, but studies suggest there are things that are known in some infants to reduce, or even stop this communication entirely. These include:

- Cessation of breastfeeding
- Infant sleeping in a separate crib not next to maternal bed
- Implementing scheduled or timed feeds and ignoring baby's cues or signals
- Ignoring night signalling, e.g. using controlled crying or other techniques. Baby may eventually accept that

his signals are ignored and thus stops communicating
- Habitual thumb, finger or pacifier sucking

When parents consult 'sleep experts' for advice on how to get their baby to achieve more adult sleep patterns, the 'expert' will attempt to show them how to get their baby to reduce or stop signalling. A good number of infants are reluctant to easily accept this and will simply call longer and louder, becoming inconsolably distressed if their signals are ignored. Stopping communication undoubtedly reduces the demand an infant makes on her caregivers. Whether this is in the best interests of the baby, in the short term (in terms of physically thriving), and in the long term (in terms of the impact of early signalling cessation), is often not considered by those who profit from teaching parents these techniques. It is presumed that increased sleep brings enough benefits to the family unit to outweigh any risks involved.

Of course, there are times when parents need support to get enough sleep to function. While most babies naturally develop a pattern that involves at least one longer unbroken sleep stretch, some infants do struggle to settle for longer than a few hours even as they get older. Many parents work outside the home after the early months, and some parents report feeling so exhausted that they feel unsafe to drive or care for their baby. However there are lots of gentle ways to naturally improve sleep, including exploring why baby is rousing so frequently.

What's even more fascinating about the complex signalling system between a baby and its mother, is that the science also suggests it isn't a one-way street. Infra-red video recordings have shown that in breastfeeding pairs (dyads) it is not always the infant who is responsible for the wake-up. Sometimes the mother signals and the baby responds. One author states:

Infants and mothers are induced to awaken by an arousal exhibited by the other (within seconds) therein creating interconnected, mutually dependent, synchronous arousals.

In short, babies and mums are programmed to regularly wake each other up. Why is this?

Dr James McKenna (recognised as the world's leading authority on maternal and infant sleep in relation to breastfeeding and SIDS) has described how frequent arousals potentially increase an infant's chance of survival, in a number of ways.

- They can protect mum's breastmilk supply, which in turn helps to protect mum from diseases such as breast and ovarian cancer.
- As discussed above, SIDS is heavily linked to arousal deficiency, so practices that prevent maternal signalling could increase risks.
- Being woken by an external factor may also improve awakening skills, which could be life-saving for the baby given that waking leads to oxygenation.

In short, Dr McKenna concludes:

Arousing is an infant's best defense against a range of potential physiological challenges.

A 2004 study explored whether there was any difference in the arousability of back-sleeping infants based on feeding method. The researchers found that during active sleep breastfed infants were significantly easier to rouse than their non-breastfed peers at 2–3 months of age.

This ties in with the research by Philip Zeskind (mentioned previously), who studied the sleep-wake patterns and heart rates of breastfed and bottle-fed newborn infants. Zeskind found that breastfed babies had lower heart rates, but that the patterns were rhythmically more complex. He wrote that in his opinion, breastfed babies developed a 'more energy-efficient and rhythmically functioning autonomic nervous system', again something key to infant arousal. In contrast, babies who were not breastfed were found 'more often in the deep-sleep state, and were overall generally less alert'.

Breastfeeding also causes babies' dopamine and adrenaline levels to rise, enhancing energy and alertness, which some suspect may also be linked to these observed behavioural differences.

Summary
- Parents of exclusively breastfed babies express concerns that their baby is behaving differently from most other babies in our society – yet most other babies receive some formula. As sleep is linked to 'good parenting' in our society, some parents might not be entirely honest about how 'well' their baby sleeps, skewing what we think of as normal.
- Premature infants have higher than typical rates of neurological problems. Several large-scale studies have found low rates of night waking and signalling among infants who were born early, suggesting communication is linked with vitality.
- Infant waking may be a problem because of the constraints that jobs and other responsibilities impose on many parents. Pre-conceived ideas about what to expect, alongside what friends and families believe is normal, can all influence whether night-waking is perceived as problematic.
- Genetics may also be linked with sleep/wake patterns and not 'habits' as some suggest.

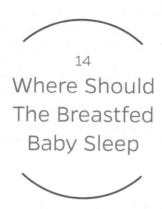

14

Where Should The Breastfed Baby Sleep

I didn't intend to cover the topic of sleep quite so much, but it's so interlinked with breastfeeding it's hard not to. One question I get asked a lot is: 'Where should my baby sleep?'

Parents are often given conflicting advice when it comes to safe sleeping, and some are given strict warnings not to share a sleep space with their baby. The official guidance from SIDS charities says that the safest place for your baby to sleep is in a cot, next to mum in her room, for the first six months.

Babies who sleep in a separate room to their parents are shown to be at up to five times the risk of SIDS than their room-sharing peers.

Babies can feed a lot at night in the early weeks and months, and a breastfeeding mum gets a huge hit of hormones that make her feel sleepy when she feeds. The biggest risk to babies is when a caregiver falls asleep sitting up holding them, on the bed and particularly the sofa. Many mums I know have admitted to unintentionally doing this, while others employ tactics such as getting up to sit in hard-backed chairs to stop themselves nodding off.

Is it any surprise that mums are driven to reduce night feeds? Mums with babies that are difficult to settle in their own space are often quickly exhausted by retrieving and returning the baby, which puts them at increased risk of unintentionally falling asleep.

Despite the fact that most parents do not plan to sleep with their baby, on any given night a fifth of all UK babies spend at least part of the night sleeping with one or both of their parents. If we pick apart the studies (including separating SIDS and suffocation, which are of course two entirely different events), the majority (although not all) bed-sharing deaths happen when:

- Parents consume alcohol, tobacco or drugs or are excessively tired.
- Parents fall asleep with the baby on a sofa (these are usually counted as bed-sharing deaths). There are a number of proposed mechanisms; from unintentionally holding baby for a long period that restricts oxygen levels, for example tucked in the crook of arm with head slightly tipped forward, to suffocation.
- Baby is placed prone (tummy down), especially on soft mattresses or when swaddled.
- Mum accidentally falls asleep breastfeeding sitting up: if her breasts are large and she slumps forward a sleeping baby can get trapped underneath. She (or any other caregiver at risk of falling asleep sitting up) can also drop the baby, or they may become wedged.
- Parents did not plan to share a sleep space with their baby and yet did so (e.g. they unexpectedly brought baby into their bed).
- Baby becomes wedged in a gap, perhaps between the mattress and a wall.

- Mum is not breastfeeding.
- Baby was between parents/next to another adult or child.
- Baby is placed near or on top of pillows.
- Baby is near or under duvet, pillows or other soft furnishings or toys.
- Baby is swaddled (this risk is also associated with cot-sleeping).

Some experts argue that making your sleep space safe – with baby lying next to you to feed (well away from any pillows, duvets and covering them with their own blanket) – is safer overall if mum unintentionally falls asleep. There is an informative website called ISIS (Infant Sleep Information Service) that Unicef and other organisations consider reputable, which discusses this in more detail.

Another option that some feel more comfortable with is a side-car crib/cot, sometimes called a co-sleeper. This is a cot that has three sides, while the fourth attaches to the bed next to mum (although often the missing side can be replaced if you're not in bed next to the baby). This arrangement can make retrieving and returning baby to his own space much easier than if he is in a standalone Moses basket or cot.

What's important is that baby and mum are together. Dr McKenna's research shows that babies sleeping just 10 feet away from their mothers breastfed 50–70 per cent less. These findings were reproduced by Professor Helen Ball and her colleagues, who showed that bedsharing babies and bed and side-car crib sleepers breastfed more frequently than infants in standalone cots just a few feet further away.

If moving infants away from mum impacts on signalling and in turn breastfeeding rates, what else could it affect? The first information I ever read on this subject was a personal experiment undertaken by Dr Sears, who explains:

In 1992 we set up equipment in our bedroom to study eight-week-old Lauren's breathing while she slept in two different arrangements. One night Lauren and Martha slept together in the same bed, as they were used to doing. The next night, Lauren slept alone in our bed and Martha slept in an adjacent room. Lauren was wired to a computer that recorded her electrocardiogram, her breathing movements, the airflow from her nose, and her blood oxygen level. The instrumentation was painless and didn't appear to disturb her sleep.

A technician and I observed and recorded the information. The data was analyzed by computer and interpreted by a pediatric pulmonologist who was 'blind' to the situation – that is, he didn't know whether the data he was analyzing came from the shared-sleeping or the solo-sleeping arrangement.

Our study revealed that Lauren breathed better when sleeping next to Martha than when sleeping alone. Her breathing and her heart rate were more regular during shared sleep, and there were fewer 'dips', low points in respiration and blood oxygen from stop-breathing episodes. On the night Lauren slept with Martha, there were no dips in her blood oxygen. On the night Lauren slept alone, there were 132 dips. The results were similar in a second infant, whose parents generously allowed us into their bedroom.

A 2011 study explored heart-rate variability in two-day-old sleeping babies for one hour each during skin-to-skin contact with mother and alone in a cot next to the mother's bed. The researchers found that sleep cycling, which means an even distribution between active and quiet sleep phases (and is considered desirable behaviour in newborns) was mostly absent in separated babies. In the 6 of 16 babies that did show some quiet sleep when separated, it was shorter and shallower.

The idea that a baby's breathing may be influenced by external sources isn't a new idea. An old study from the 1980s showed that even premature infants sought contact with a source of rhythmic stimulation that reflected their own breathing rhythm, in this case a teddy with a 'heartbeat'. The infants showed greater amounts of quiet sleep than babies who slept with a teddy without a heartbeat. Other biological studies suggest that these cues act as 'hidden' stimuli, by which the young of other mammals time their next breath.

Dr McKenna has explored this area too, and looked at the impact mum's expelled carbon dioxide (CO_2) might have on her baby in a bed-sharing situation. While prolonged high levels of CO_2 are dangerous, he feels short bursts may serve a different purpose. One study found that a 10-second burst of 7 per cent CO_2 acted as a 'powerful respiratory stimulant' for premature infants. There are very few studies, but one with adult participants found that 2-minute challenges with 15 per cent CO_2 produced constant increases in ventilation.

What's even more interesting are Dr McKenna's observations of how often mothers check their babies, which usually consisted of touching rather than just looking. The study didn't find any significant difference in the total amount of time overall that bed-sharing mothers spent checking their infants relative to mothers of cot-sleeping infants, but the frequency of checking was much greater among the bed-sharing group than the cot-sleeping group.

These more frequent checks did not always result in full arousals and small patting movements were seen despite the appearance of sleep.

The suggestion is that breastfeeding mothers are 'tuned in' to the presence of their baby, even when they are asleep.

Dr McKenna's work has also highlighted the following:

- Both non-ventilated blankets and mums and babies snuggled together under covers can create a pocket of air around the baby's head which may allow increased and potentially dangerous levels of CO_2 to accumulate.
- The more frequent arousals observed when bed-sharing may contribute to preventing high levels of CO_2; arousal prompts breathing and oxygenation.
- All but one breastfeeding baby slept on their back or side. The one baby who slept prone was placed in that position by his mother.
- Babies spent most of their time with their head turned to face mum, unless they were placed prone, which appeared to hinder this natural gravitation.
- Previous studies have shown that back-sleeping babies also turn their heads to the side where the scent of breastmilk is present.
- The vast majority of mums adopted what is now widely recognised as the standard bed-sharing position. Mum is side-lying to face baby, knees pulled up, one arm folded under her head.

The distance between the faces of mum and baby for the majority of dyads was less than 20cm.

Dr McKenna concludes that breastfeeding mother-infant pairs exhibit increased sensitivities and responses to each other while sleeping, and those sensitivities offer the infant protection from overlay. However, bottle-feeding infants should lie alongside the mother in a crib or bassinet, not in the same bed.

Certain medical groups, including some members of the American Academy of Pediatrics (though not necessarily the majority), argue that bed-sharing should be eliminated altogether and some professionals believe that it can never be made safe.

Sleep facts

- Babies kept close to mum tend to feed more frequently, which establishes a good milk supply and increases breastfeeding success rates. In turn, keeping baby close makes frequent feeding easier for parents and is shown in several studies to increase breastfeeding success rates.
- Babies who breastfeed on cue day and night are less likely to become habitual thumb, finger or pacifier suckers, which may hinder their signalling and reduce night feeds (and in turn affect baby's weight gain).
- Rousing has significant benefits for both mum and baby, with healthier infants signalling more frequently.
- One study found that 25 per cent of all babies had not regularly slept from 10pm to 6am by the age of one year.
- At 12 months over half of all babies wake at night.
- Popular beliefs about when babies should be 'sleeping through the night' are based on studies conducted in the 1950s and 1960s on groups of formula-fed babies. As a result nearly a third of parents feel their child has 'sleep problems'.
- Babies wake more in the second half of the first year than the first. While in one study 71 per cent of babies had 'slept through the night' on at least one occasion by three months of age, many of these reported more frequent waking in the 4 to 12-month period.

- It is not until after 24 months that regular night waking (requiring attention) becomes much less common.
- Infant sleep studies highlight the wide range in total hours slept by infants of the same age. Despite books often stating that there are ideal or optimum sleep durations, this isn't what evidence suggests. For example, in one study the average total sleeping time for 4-month-old infants ranged from 11 to 19 hours; over the course of the six-day study, individual infants showed wide variations in their sleeping times with a range as great as 12 hours.
- Babies sleeping alone in cots can also suffer SIDS (previously called 'cot-death').

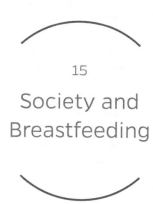

15

Society and Breastfeeding

Aside from the physical ability to lactate, the desire to breastfeed and the need for good support, there is another key factor that helps determine whether women breastfeed successfully. How supportive society as a whole is of breastfeeding is also shown to have a significant influence on outcome.

I'm sure many people would argue that in the UK we have a breastfeeding-friendly society. Plenty of shops provide breastfeeding rooms, and sometimes mums who are not breastfeeding report that they are the ones who feel like everyone is judging them. However, a quick scan of the headlines shows how mums are still sometimes asked to stop breastfeeding in public, or to cover themselves up to ensure they feed 'modestly'. Celebrities like Jeremy Clarkson have likened lactating to urinating in public and Dr Christian Jessen, a well-known 'anti-obesity' campaigner, used the terms 'breastfeeding militants' and 'breastapo' on Twitter, despite the fact that not breastfeeding is directly linked to an increased risk of obesity.

Imagine if these people had made similar comments, but the words 'breastfeeding' or 'milk' were replaced with terms denoting race, religion or sexuality. It would be completely unacceptable. But while it's not politically correct to name-call most minority groups in our society, breastfeeders seem to be fair game.

Women are also told they should express and use a bottle when out and about, and we see polls asking whether breastfeeding in public is acceptable – even when we have laws that clearly state that mothers can breastfeed anywhere that they are entitled to be.

If our society is anti-bottle and pro-breast, where are the bottle-feeding covers? When did someone last suggest that bottle-feeding was sexual, or that baby should stop having a teat once they have teeth, because continuing to bottle-feed beyond that point was purely for the mother's benefit? One mum said:

> *I have been called an exhibitionist, disgusting, perverted, accused of harming my child, told to go hide in a bathroom/closet, and alienated from family situations because of breastfeeding.*

An NCT survey of 1,200 women found 65 per cent didn't intend to even try breastfeeding in public, because they felt too self-conscious about people staring at them.

The irony of a culture that embraces scantily-clad females in almost every other context, from adverts to music videos, but recoils at a mum breastfeeding, is surely obvious. But why can't breasts be multifunctional, when so many other body parts are? Mouths can talk, eat, vomit *and* kiss – why can't breasts be both sexual and functional? That this is peculiar to our culture is clear when you consider that in Japan, for example, the nape of the neck is considered far more sexual than a breast. We're influenced by what we see around us every day and the messages the media reinforce.

In the UK we have been a bottle-feeding culture since around the time of the Second World War. Since then, although many believe we are more liberal than ever – this only really applies to the sexualisation of women's bodies, rather than when women choose to use their bodies to nurture their young. Many people today can *only* relate to breasts in a sexual context, forgetting that as mammals our mammary glands exist primarily to produce milk for our young. Anything else is an added bonus. Whereas many of the older generation can remember being squeezed up against a breastfeeding mum on a bus or train, many younger people are now conditioned to seeing babies drinking from bottles, especially in public.

Breastfeeding in public

There's an interesting discrepancy between how acceptable mums feel breastfeeding in public is, and the attitude of the general public. A 2015 poll by Public Health England found that mothers were anxious about feeding in public, with 1 in 5 (21 per cent) feeling that the general public didn't want them to do it. A huge 60 per cent of mums tried to hide the fact they were feeding and more than a third felt embarrassed or uncomfortable. In contrast, the same poll found that nearly three quarters of the general public polled supported public breastfeeding and *didn't* find it offensive.

A poll from the Irish Department of Health, Social Services and Public Safety also from 2015, reported that only 4 per cent of those surveyed found breastfeeding offensive and distasteful. 87 per cent supported public breastfeeding and over 70 per cent felt it should be protected by law.

So breastfeeding mums feel self-conscious and judged, and formula or bottle-feeding mums feel exactly the same. Mums are worried about being judged *however* they feed their baby.

The impact of bottle-feeding culture

When most mums don't breastfeed, or don't breastfeed for long, other people in society may undermine a mum's efforts without even knowing they're doing so, because basic awareness of breastfeeding norms has been lost. If the majority breastfeed, friends and relatives can share tips and tricks, with the underlying expectation that mum will succeed. People would understand that breastfeeding can take time to become established. Nobody expects to get in a vehicle for the first time and then join the nearest motorway; we all understand that it can take patience and time to fully develop the coordination and skills required to deftly pull off a three-point turn.

In a society that has lost valuable skills like recognising the earliest signs of a problem and knowing how best to help, a common answer to almost every problem is to switch to formula feeding. It's sold as convenient because others can feed the baby and give mum a break. It's easy to understand, it's a fixed product and so set amounts and a routine can be established (something else mums today are told is essential).

However, the reality of safe formula preparation at 3am is anything but easy, and having to tote bottles, powder and water everywhere is hardly convenient. But if that's what you perceive as normal and those around you can't help you with breastfeeding, what can you do?

Other questions we have to ask are what does our society value most – health or aesthetics, attachment or independence? How quickly babies become 'self-soothers', and how rapidly after birth mothers can achieve their 'pre-baby body' have become markers of success. If a celebrity can attend an important function and look like she's never given birth, it's a double whammy. Dads are rarely subject to such scrutiny. There are no features online or in the media giving dads tips on how to 'have it all', so they can fit in plucking their eyebrows, folding laundry and a quick workout for those chunky thighs before an afternoon in the office. Slummy mummy, yummy mummy, work just enough but not too much mummy – what was that about 'girl power'?

Then there's the insidious, underlying fear that babies not pushed or encouraged to become independent will become needy. That if they sleep next to you they will never want to sleep alone, if you carry them they will never want to be put down. This idea is so ingrained, that I was once asked whether I was concerned that my premature, not even 2.2kg (5lb) baby in a sling might become 'clingy'.

Independence

In stark contrast to our cultural fears about clingy children, what studies show, time and time again, is the exact opposite: in fact, responsive, loving care drives secure attachment and thus independent behaviour.

Dr Eleanor Maccoby, a renowned child development researcher, completed a study exploring the response time of parents and longer-term outcomes. She noted that babies who were responded to rapidly grew up to be the most independent and curious toddlers. She concluded that babies know how to get people to fulfil their needs – they cry and then they smile when someone comes. Furthermore, toddlers know how to explore the world – they use their loved ones as a safe base from which to explore.

All makes logical sense, even from an adult's perspective. If you're in a relationship with someone loving and caring, does feeling secure make you dependent and clingy? In fact, if we look at human nature the reverse is true; people who feel insecure are far more likely to seek attention and reassurance that they are loved. Most of you will have heard the old adage 'treat them mean, keep them keen'.

Cognitive dissonance

Another problem we have when breastfeeding is not the norm in society, is that infant feeding decisions can easily trigger a state called 'cognitive dissonance'. This is the term given to the feelings we can experience when we hold two views that conflict with each other. Humans like consistency in their thoughts and behaviour and find the feelings of discomfort that result from holding two opposing views unpleasant. As a result we are motivated to rationalise the situation as quickly as possible.

Cognitive dissonance can be triggered by almost anything, so when it comes to parenting there's lots of potential. We know that certain situations trigger more intense dissonance than others. For example, if the decision is important (or perceived as such); if something is learnt retrospectively but the opportunity to change the decision or outcome has passed; or if we felt forced into the initial decision rather than it being a free choice.

Again this makes logical sense, and again we see this in practice. Let's take baby rice, historically the first food for many babies. More recent evidence has suggested that it's probably not the best choice for babies; in fact it's probably not even a good choice. How do mums at different stages respond to the new information?

- A mum who is pregnant may file that away as worth exploring more when the time for solids comes.

- A mum about to introduce solids may start searching immediately for more information, current guidelines and recommendations.
- A mum currently using baby rice may either decide not to use it again, or she may have an emotional response, such as feeling upset, angry or guilty.
- A mum who has used baby rice for previous babies may either be uninterested in the new information, or have a similar emotional response to those currently using baby rice.

The mums most likely to respond with dissonance to the information are those in the last two groups.

Whether you feed your child baby rice is probably seen as a pretty insignificant decision compared to the decision about what type of milk to feed your baby. In a society in which many women don't meet their breastfeeding goals, it's easy to see that a huge group of mothers are likely to experience cognitive dissonance.

When it comes to decision-making, we are also more likely to lean towards our original belief than we are to change our behaviour (although the latter is possible). So in the above situation, a mum may simply argue that she uses or used it, and her children are fine. This is the most typical response if a mild level of dissonance is triggered.

Next we have a moderate response; this may start out as basic denial, but if the person is experiencing more intense feelings of discomfort, it can prompt them to look for more information to support their original belief. In the example above, the answer may be to search for information promoting the consumption of baby rice. What's more, we know that people in this state actively avoid material that would support the new, proposed theory. There is rarely a balanced approach or a full re-evaluation of the evidence (although of course, not everyone experiences dissonance, and some will be able to look objectively at the evidence).

Intense dissonance occurs when the person can no longer convince themselves of their original belief. The only way out of this distress is to accept the new information.

In our society, huge groups of people have the internal belief that nowadays formula is nearly as good as breastmilk. They look around and see relatives, friends and family who were formula-fed, as were their babies, and they are all 'fine'. We can see this reflected in surveys, in which the majority will simultaneously agree with the statements 'breastfeeding has health benefits' and 'formula doesn't have health risks'.

Referring to benefits as though they're something extra special, over and above our perception of 'normal', doesn't appear to trigger cognitive dissonance in the same way that discussion of risks does. Because of this, much recent debate has focused on whether we should ensure our language does not trigger dissonance. This is another topic in itself, but we should note that successful health campaigns such as smoking cessation and drink-driving prevention often deliver a consistent, hard-hitting message – designed to initially trigger intense dissonance and ultimately acceptance.

When it comes to infant feeding, it's a ridiculously hard political landscape to negotiate. You only have to look at the heated and explosive public exchanges on the subject, from Jamie Oliver to Adele, to see that. This creates a challenge for those providing breastfeeding support, who are often addressing an audience made up of people from different backgrounds, who have all had different experiences and who hold different pre-conceived ideas.

We also have to acknowledge that some mums just don't want to breastfeed. There could be any number of reasons why this is, from the really complex, deep and personal, to a simple, deep-seated belief that breastfeeding doesn't really matter. If this mum then finds herself feeling like she has to breastfeed (for whatever reason) – again she's likely to experience dissonance. Perhaps this is why sharing evidence-based information about infant feeding is perceived by some as 'pressure to breastfeed'?

The impact of a formula-feeding culture on breastfeeding support

The other problem with a mainly formula-feeding society is that it affects the quality of breastfeeding support mums receive. It is easy to get stuck in a cycle of poor support leading to low rates and reliance on substitutes, which leads to more poor support, and so on.

If we hold the basic belief that there is an easily accessible alternative that is nearly as good as breastmilk, then why bother trying to resolve more complex breastfeeding problems? Mums often tell me that this really perplexes some of those around them; they're often asked why they don't just give formula. Furthermore, if we don't have the skills to help parents to succeed, even if the majority of people want to breastfeed, there may not be the support in place for them to do so.

If we lose sight of what is and isn't normal for a breastfed infant, because we're comparing their behaviour to formula-fed babies, sometimes old wives' tales replace facts. Although we can learn the technicalities of lactation, how milk is produced and what baby does when suckling to transfer it effectively, what can be much more difficult to develop are the practical skills to evaluate the quality of milk transfer. Identifying good attachment during an actual breastfeed is difficult if you've never actually seen many people breastfeed well.

This is the situation in the UK at the moment. I'm frequently surprised to see NHS infant feeding material or posters showing babies poorly attached to the breast. Many mothers I see have been told that their baby is feeding 'fine', and yet when I work with them on attachment they can't understand why the people who tried to support them earlier didn't have the same knowledge.

We have also lost the subtle skills of reading baby's body language, facial expressions, gestures and sounds. Babies tell us almost everything we need to know, but we need to translate this – and if formula-fed and breastfed babies communicate differently (which evidence suggests they do), we have another layer of complexity to navigate.

I recently supported a mum who was trying to latch her fussing baby to the breast. He was giving strong, clear wind signals and so we discussed holding him upright for a moment to see if he needed to release a burp. Indeed he did; three giant belches before settling down to his feed. Mum reported that several people she had seen had watched a feed and told her baby had reflux, or maybe a dairy intolerance, and that she should try infant Gaviscon and cutting out dairy. In fact he gulped lots of air at the start of his feed, which soon caused discomfort. Later the baby began squirming again, indicating discomfort at the bottom end this time. I showed the parents how to gently release the trapped gas, at which point he (spectacularly) demonstrated the effectiveness of the technique, to the extent that it could probably be heard next door, before promptly falling asleep.

I am not a witch, as this couple initially claimed. Often breastfeeding support in the community is focused on a checklist and trying to achieve formula-feeding norms. People are busy, and often don't have time to sit and watch the subtleties of feeding; often it's a weight check, ask about nipple pain and done.

Breastfeeding supporters need to be able to tell the difference between a baby wriggling with wind, and one who is doing so to increase the flow of the milk. A baby who grabs, squirms and pulls can be doing so for any number of reasons. If we can't work it out, we risk incorrectly diagnosing babies with conditions like 'silent reflux' and medicating them accordingly. Some babies do suffer from reflux for a medical reason, but some are refluxing as a direct result of the way they feed. Others aren't refluxing at all; they're trying to communicate something else entirely.

I also wonder whether, because we are trying to increase breastfeeding rates, some panic if a mum says she has a problem. It's as though if we agree things aren't 'optimum', she may throw her arms in the air immediately and quit.

Recently I took a call from a mum who had stopped breastfeeding weeks ago, but was having problems with bottles. When breastfeeding her baby had been attached hour after hour; when she eventually did take him off, he still wasn't satisfied and needed the extra bottle-feed anyway. Mum had searched online and been told by several different people that it was normal for breastfed babies to want to feed all the time. Quite understandably, the mum didn't feel this was sustainable, and she made the difficult decision to stop breastfeeding. Isn't there a risk that mums like this may believe that some women must just be super-tough to get through it?

I see the same problem regularly online and often from passionate breastfeeding supporters. A mum describes a picture of baby feeding constantly day and night, yet the baby may only gain small amounts of weight in return for the hours put in. Mum's nipples might be a bit sore, but again they may not. Is this normal, she asks? The correct answer is that without knowing more, it's impossible to tell. Without knowing the history and asking lots more questions, nobody can really have any idea whether it's normal establishment of feeding, or an early indication that some support may be needed. An ideal response will give details of where mum can get more help, be that online or in person, and perhaps some tips and tricks to try in the meantime.

However, the replies I often see fall into two different groups:

1. Wear baby in a sling, co-sleep and feed, feed, feed on demand; it's all entirely normal. Sometimes mums add stories about their own babies who barely gained weight but were fine, or report that they survived 17 hours per day of feeding and even now, at a year, their baby still wakes 42 times in the night. It's normal! But is it?

   Sometimes of course the reassurance may be warranted: if baby is having a temporary blip and a fussy spell, or just being a newborn, then sharing survival tips and tricks between mums is hugely beneficial. Sometimes parents do have unrealistic expectations and their baby is in fact feeding to a normal healthy pattern.

   However, sometimes parents are describing what could potentially be an ongoing problem. Sometimes mum can't sustain the demand even if she does all the above – and even then, her gut feeling may tell her something isn't quite right. Sometimes weight gain isn't small, but huge – yet baby still seems to be constantly signalling for food.

   It's not uncommon for this gut feeling, conflicting with what she's being told, to cause mum to feel as though she is imagining or creating a problem when one doesn't really exist. Some mums are really apologetic about needing a consultation, and say that their problems are probably normal and they just need to 'get used to it' or 'hold baby a bit differently'.

2. Just give formula. I couldn't breastfeed and my baby is fine, we had a different baby from the moment we introduced that first bottle, so contented and slept like a dream and so on and so forth.

The problem is that there can be so many subtle variations between one situation and another, that these one-size-fits-all responses are unhelpful. Consider for a moment that to qualify to sit the exam to become an Internationally Board Certified Lactation Consultant, 1,000 hours of clinical practice are required. Babies and bodies are unique, and as such we can't base effective support on the anecdotal experience of others. Early identification of problems leads to the easiest resolution – but mums can often be left confused about what is and isn't normal, whether their problems can be resolved, and whose advice to listen to.

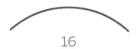

16

The Impact of Formula Marketing - Breastfeeding, Guilt and Judgement

Globally, the marketing of formula is recognised as enough of a threat to breastfeeding that in 1981 the World Health Organisation ratified the International Code of Marketing of Breastmilk Substitutes. This document recommends that all countries should introduce legislation to ban the advertising of formula milk. In the UK first infant milk (milk intended to replace breastmilk in the first six months) cannot be advertised or promoted for sale by means of special offers, vouchers, discounts or promotions.

It's important to clarify that the Code does not prohibit a permanent price reduction on infant formula. If a manufacturer currently sells a tin for £10, they are legally allowed to reduce this to £5 if this is a permanent change. The restrictions mean they can't promote the product with a temporary reduced price, marketing display or any other technique designed to induce sales.

I find that in reality many parents don't believe this, and are often convinced that they've seen a formula advert on

TV. In fact what UK consumers see are adverts for follow-on milk, a product that appeared on the market shortly after the legislation restricting the advertising of first milk came into force. It is virtually identical to first infant milk – except that it contains (unnecessary) additional iron – but it is labelled as suitable from six months to get around the regulations.

It's not unusual for parents to ask why the Code really matters, as they think that adverts simply inform consumers about the different products out there so they can decide what to buy. People often think that if someone wants to breastfeed, a TV advert isn't going to make any difference at all. However, adverts don't simply let us know that a product exists; they aim to sell it to us. Companies spend tens of thousands of pounds on advertising campaigns because research shows that we are all – whether we like it or not! – influenced by advertising.

A 2006 report found that UK formula manufacturers spent around £20 per baby born promoting formula, while the government spent approximately 14 pence per baby born promoting breastfeeding. It's anything but a level playing field.

Breastfeeding rates in Norway in the 1970s were comparable to those in the UK today. However, Norway banned all advertising of artificial formula milk completely. They also increased maternity leave to a year at 80 per cent of salary, and when mums do return to work they're given an hour's expressing break daily. Today 98 per cent of Norwegian women start out breastfeeding, and 90 per cent are still nursing four months later.

In the last 30 years there has been a seismic shift in how people access and share information. The internet connects users around the globe; journal abstracts are accessed within a couple of clicks and virtual strangers discuss the merits of almost every aspect of parenting. Rather than parents relying on health professionals, books or off-the-shelf magazines, the latest generation has access to raw data like never before. This carries both risks and benefits. The biggest problem is that after reading a relatively small amount or with a little experience, everyone is an expert – or at least they think they are. This is known as the 'Dunning-Kruger effect'.

Sometimes rapid sharing is hugely beneficial as it's estimated that most new evidence takes around five years to reach healthcare systems at a working level. At other times, a little bit of knowledge can be a dangerous thing.

In terms of infant feeding, the availability of information presents parents with a significant dilemma. Research overwhelmingly tells us that how we feed our babies matters, yet we have a population where the vast majority are not breastfeeding.

As we've discussed, presenting breastfeeding as something 'beneficial', 'extra' and offering more than formula doesn't really work. People generally don't strive for 'best', they settle for average or good enough. Discussing breastfeeding in terms of risks triggers cognitive dissonance, which may provoke change, or extreme hostility.

What mothers feel about information that is shared on infant feeding is often, in my experience, a whole range of emotions, based on their own situation:

- Denial: My kids were formula-fed and are fine so I think the study is nonsense.
- Anger: Some of us can't breastfeed; think about how you make us feel when you share these studies!
- Interest: I'm pregnant and had no idea breastfeeding was linked with this.
- Happiness: I'm so glad I stuck at breastfeeding when I read things like this.
- Guilt: I have only just stopped feeling guilty I couldn't breastfeed and didn't need to see this.

If a single article can provoke all these responses, what should we do?

Another problem is that lack of effective support effectively means lack of choice. Yet this is cyclic: if we don't acknowledge breastfeeding's importance, there is no incentive to improve support. If we were to properly acknowledge the risks of not breastfeeding, it would be far harder for healthcare systems to continue to be unsupportive.

Demand drives change – yet we are in a cycle where those who make up the biggest numbers and are most affected (formula users) are the most loyal to formula. It's often those who are breastfeeding who are most vocal about demanding improvements – right before they get accused of being militant.

So despite the pro-breastfeeding message many mothers receive, little improvement has occurred in terms of tangible support. Thanks to budget cuts many areas are now offering significantly less support than they were ten years ago. The Department of Health has scrapped all the promotional materials they used to send out for Breastfeeding Awareness Week, and they've scrapped the Infant Feeding Survey that gave us vital information about the rates of breastfeeding and formula feeding, and about how and when babies start solids. Despite its huge significance for the health of the nation, breastfeeding seems to be at the bottom of the list of priorities.

The media *really* struggle with all this when it comes to reporting. Ultimately, the newspaper editors know that the majority of their readers use formula – yet they also want and need to report actual news. Recently a leading UK newspaper published a breastfeeding article with the comment 'Here's another study to make women feel like failures'. Surely it's society that is contributing to why women feel like failures, not the scientific research?

Mums who observe this often become angry and sometimes become the most vocal pro-breastfeeding supporters. They want to prevent other mums experiencing what they did, and share the knowledge they have gleaned. They may have had problems breastfeeding themselves, but they now understand why. However, these breastfeeding advocates can quickly find themselves labelled the 'breastfeeding mafia', despite the fact that they were once on the opposite side of the fence and using formula.

Other mums want to share the joy they've experienced once they've finally cracked breastfeeding, often after a difficult start and against the odds. Yet doing so will undoubtedly result in them being considered smug by mums who have had a different journey.

The wide range of emotions mothers feel is the basis for what the media calls the 'mummy wars'. It starts with the marketing message that 'breast is best', a strategy heavily pushed by formula companies.

Think about buying a chicken at the supermarket: you have value chickens, standard chickens and free-range/organic chickens. In reality, free-range or organic chickens have really just had a normal chicken life. A standard chicken is anything but standard, unless we call living in a tiny cramped crate with no access to the outside world 'normal'. So really our free-range/organic chicken should just be chicken. Others should be 'caged chickens' or 'honestly, we've had a pretty dire life' chickens, but I think most people can see that these wouldn't be top sellers.

What the marketing bods do to get around this is to elevate the norm to 'finest' or 'organic', which neatly allows a substandard product to take the label 'standard'. Marketing companies know from years of market research that most people consider 'standard' to be 'good enough'; so much so that they sell millions more standard chickens than 'finest' ones, even if there isn't much of a price difference.

Once you're aware of this marketing method you can spot it all around you on a daily basis. Tomatoes ripened on the vine (where they grow) are 'speciality', whereas those picked early, ripened en route rather than in the sun, which resemble watery balls of tasteless mush, are just 'tomatoes'.

You're probably wondering what on earth supermarket shopping, chickens, tomatoes and customer faith have to do with the mummy wars, but it's important to understand this strategy as it's central to formula marketing.

Once overwhelming research demonstrated that formula-fed babies were at greater risk of health problems, it became impossible to continue marketing formula as superior to breastmilk. Instead the formula companies adopted the technique described above, elevating breastmilk to 'best' – the equivalent of 'finest' or 'organic' – thus allowing formula to take the 'standard' tag. Elevating breastmilk to 'best' means it is associated with words including 'perfect' and 'optimum'. Marketers know that as a society we are drilled in the art of moderation.

It's not uncommon for me to hear expectant mothers say that they are going to try breastfeeding, but if they need to use some formula they're not going to be 'extreme' about it. This is perfect for the formula companies, which are more than happy to be seen as 'standard', 'normal' or 'average'. The companies are even happy to provide support for mums to breastfeed, because in doing so they can emphasise just how hard breastfeeding is.

Once the message we are all pushing is that 'breast is best', where does that leave mums who aren't breastfeeding? It is easy for mums in that position to feel inferior and judged, and to perceive others who are 'giving the best' as smug. This is a notion the formula companies embrace, because any divide between parents hinders the effective sharing of information and strengthens their market. It also allows them to step in as the support for these 'not best' parents, with adverts such as 'you're doing great' – in other words, don't feel bad about that whole breastfeeding thing.

Baby Milk Action, a non-profit organisation which aims to end avoidable suffering caused by inappropriate infant feeding, is part of a global network called IBFAN (the International Baby Food Action Network). In 2016 they alerted the public to the webpage of a marketing company. It read as follows:

> *Futureproof were briefed to create a deeper relationship between SMA and mums, and take the relationship from 'necessary product' to 'trusted brand and partner'.*
>
> *SMA needed to deepen the relationship they had with mums, and create a relationship that went beyond the product.*
>
> *From our research, we discovered that the main thing that mums wanted was reassurance. Reassurance that at this incredibly tricky, emotional, and daunting time, they were making the right decisions and doing ok. Particularly around the delicate, emotional, and controversial subject of breastfeeding and weaning.*

As a result, SMA's next campaign had the tagline 'You're doing great'. The advert runs like this:

Visual: A mum holding a bottle and trying to soothe baby during the night, a mum realising just before she puts baby in the pushchair he has a dirty nappy, a baby throwing food which hits her, a mum struggling to collapse a pushchair before abandoning it.

Voiceover: *'You don't have to sit an exam, you've no*

experience, but the job's still yours.'

Visual: Pulling SMA tin from cupboard causes bottles to fall out, then a dad pulling faces at baby to entertain him while mum and baby look on bemused.

Voiceover: *'You learn as you go, doing whatever it takes.'*

The advertiser has let the audience know that they understand and relate to them – we've all been there with the dirty nappy just before leaving the house, or on the receiving end of food lobbing. It makes us laugh and builds an affinity with the viewer.

Visual: Can of SMA follow on milk and mum making up a bottle, then her sitting back and relaxing as baby has a feed.

Voiceover: *'At SMA our follow-on milk is supported by 90 years' experience.'*

The key message is that this is a product supported by lots of research. It's no coincidence that the visuals shift from a struggling mum to a relaxing mum when the product and its use are displayed.

Visual: Mum relaxing in a bath, before finding she's sat on a rubber duck, which she tosses out and goes back to relaxing.

Voiceover: *'And over the years we've really got to know mums, and take it from us, you're doing great'.*

This is all designed to reinforce the message that SMA is an authority on the subject of infant feeding, and that they really relate to you, right before delivering the message they knew parents wanted to hear: 'You're doing great'. Throughout a catchy soundtrack about unconditional love is playing.

Slow hand clap for the genius marketing team; it's brilliant in terms of marketing isn't it? And it worked well in practice:

> *The results were outstanding and immediate. Within six months, the brand increased levels of interactivity with mums, and dramatically shifted the perceptions of*

SMA to a more 'caring' and 'supportive' space.

But perhaps the most encouraging result has been that commercially the brand moved from number three in market to number two within six months, and is now pushing to regain the number one spot.

What's more, the price charged for a can of formula means that the company's profits can more than cover the market research and the resulting adverts, meaning that mothers (and it is mothers, as fathers rarely give a hoot whether a marketing bod thinks they're doing fine) in effect pay to be reassured that they're doing great. Formula milk could be considerably cheaper if the companies spent less on advertising it.

The pressure to 'parent perfectly' generates behaviour that becomes divisive. If you feel insecure and vulnerable, you present a front of certainty to hide it. Parents with similar experiences often group together for support. From there the 'mummy wars' are almost self-perpetuating. If you tell people they're being judged and perceived as inferior by another group, they're prone to acting defensively in response and may attack others. Another formula company did exactly this in another advert, which suggested that mothers were all judging each other.

A large US brand released an advert called 'The Sisterhood of Motherhood', which runs for a whole two and a half minutes. This is *huge* for a commercial. It depicts extreme 'types' of mothers being hostile to each other, judging, and arguing among themselves. There is a group with prams, one with slings, working mums, cloth-nappy-using mums, yoga mums and so on, including of course breastfeeding and bottle-feeding mums. Dads are present, but despite the prams, slings and other visible differences they're all sat together, symbolising unity.

The opening line is 'Oh look, the breast police have arrived', to which the breastfeeding mums reply '100% breastfed, straight from the source'. The next mum pipes up 'Drug-free pool birth, dolphin assisted'. Next those with slings say 'You push, we cuddle, cuddling is bonding', to which a dad replies 'Helicopter mum at 12 o'clock!'. There's a comment about cloth nappies, a dig at working mums and those that stay at home and then it's back to breastfeeding: 'Some mums are too lazy to breastfeed'.

The fight threatens to get physical until, at the last moment, a pram rolls away down a hill with a baby still inside. The slow-motion camera kicks in as everyone races to catch it. When they do, there's a relieved hug and everyone starts being friends. On the screen the following words appear: 'No matter what our beliefs, we are parents first…'

The advert was widely shared on social media. Many thought it was a feminist concept – women choose, they should be supported not judged. Absolutely. However, the reverse is true and it's actually a brilliant example of advertising that undermines women rather than supporting them. From referencing the 'breast police', to calling those who don't breastfeed 'lazy', the not-so-subtle implication is that mothers are judging each other about feeding decisions. The advert also neatly presents feeding as another 'belief', comparable to any other parenting choice, and it effectively silences women.

Who wants to be perceived as judgemental or extreme? Who wants to think they've made another person feel 'guilty' or 'bad' because of a choice they've made? Who wants to be the woman in the advert thinking she's superior? We know, as do the advert makers, that women want reassurance that they're doing well.

I ran a quick poll on my Facebook page to ask readers if

hearing about judgement and the 'mummy wars' as a result of this advert had affected how they shared news or articles related to infant feeding on social media. Even I was surprised at the results.

From just over 365 replies, a massive 50 per cent reported that they were less likely to share something related to infant feeding, with only 7 per cent more likely to do so – that's a 43 per cent reduction in material shared online. What's more, a further 17 per cent no longer share *any* infant feeding related material, while only a quarter of all respondents felt their sharing was not influenced by this cultural shift and continued to share as they always did.

A few added comments like:
- *I share but with context so that mothers hopefully feel less judged.*
- *I share with consideration as some friends chose to formula feed. I won't share anything that I feel will be divisive.*
- *Sometimes I share more things to raise awareness and sometimes I think twice about potential arguments before sharing.*
- *I still share but I sometimes worry if by doing so I am offending my formula feeding friends.*

That's surely a hugely successful campaign if your aim is to reduce the amount of material out there that might help mums to successfully breastfeed or encourage them to want to do so. Every mum that breastfeeds successfully is one less customer for the companies. When billions of pounds of profit are at stake, do we really expect them to play nicely?

Mothers are often angry that they've been failed, and of course some people just like to argue or belittle others –

men and women can be rude, insensitive and unkind. But to pretend that the offensive minority accurately represent what the vast majority of people think is ridiculous. In my experience mothers usually judge themselves far more harshly than others do.

Mums who bottlefeed in public often say they feel judged by breastfeeders, yet when you sit down and unpick their feelings it turns out that the breastfeeder didn't do anything to suggest she was judging the other mother. She just sat there feeding (probably trying to be 'discreet', as society demands).

Similarly, a breastfeeding mum may feel nervous feeding in a place where every other mum is bottle-feeding, perhaps because she has previously been told that breastfeeding is gross and should be done at home, not in public. Could she not express for when out and about? She feels just as judged, despite the fact the bottle-feeding mums are probably utterly lovely.

The 'mummy wars' is not about groups of mothers hating each other as the media would have you believe (Most mothers struggle to find time to pee without the company of a small human, let alone undertake an act of war). It's about groups of mums feeling judged because they're constantly being told its happening.

Breastfeeding matters. More than that, mothers matter. Genuinely supporting mothers who want to breastfeed, to do so for as long as they wish, could trigger a paradigm shift in UK infant feeding practices that would indeed facilitate a truly informed choice.

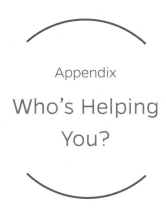

Appendix

Who's Helping You?

When it comes to breastfeeding support, parents often aren't aware of the different people that are available to help, or what their level of expertise is. In the UK mums are attended by midwives after birth and then health visitors, and currently there is a lot of variability in the quality of support given. Some are very experienced, have fed their own babies or undertaken additional training; others recycle out-of-date advice and parents sometimes report that every person they see contradicts the others.

Some areas employ an infant feeding advisor, or have an infant feeding team which is a specialist (in theory) group of practitioners who can support breastfeeding in the hospital and community. This isn't standard in all areas, however, and again there is huge variability reported across the country in terms of the skills of those employed and the satisfaction parents report when accessing these services.

There are also other people available who can help.

Peer supporter
Also called: breastfeeding peer counsellor, peer helper, mother supporter, breastfeeding buddy and breastfeeding specialist. Some areas have schemes to help mums get in touch with these supporters, and they may have an umbrella name such as 'Breast Friends' or 'Breastfeeding Buddies'. These are mums who may or may not have breastfed their own children and want to support other mums. Peer supporters complete a short training course and can work in a variety of settings in the role of a supportive, experienced and knowledgeable friend. Some are volunteers, while others are employed by the local hospital.

A peer supporter should:
- Be a well-informed friend. The role was developed because nowadays lots of mums don't know anyone who has breastfed that they can learn the basics from. A peer (and the clue is in the name) can share tips about everything from how to hold and latch baby on and the best position to wind them, to their favourite brand of breastpad.
- Discuss what is normal for a breastfed baby, covering things like growth spurts and cluster feeding.
- Help you access more specialist help should problems arise.

A peer supporter should not:
- Act in a medical capacity, assessing or examining you or your baby.
- Give advice or tell you what to do.
- Try to solve an ongoing breastfeeding concern.
- Peer supporters are a key way the NHS provides local breastfeeding support and it's great; we need lots of them. However, some areas don't employ enough (or

indeed any) people with more training or experience to whom the peer supporters can refer.

Healthcare assistant/maternity support assistant/health support worker

These health workers work alongside nurses and midwives and are sometimes known as nursing auxiliaries. No breastfeeding training or qualification is required for this role; some may have undertaken a day or two of breastfeeding support training. Despite this lack of training these workers regularly provide breastfeeding support in some areas, particularly in units where the midwives are in high demand and don't have as much time to sit with mothers as they would like.

Breastfeeding counsellor

Also called: La Leche League Leader, breastfeeding consultant, breastfeeding supporter. These are mums or health professionals who, in addition to completing the peer support training, have exclusively breastfed their own baby for at least 6–9 months, until there was a nutritional need for other foods (i.e., about the middle of the first year for the healthy, full-term baby) and completed further training. This may be done by distance learning and attending local support groups, or via meetings and in-person depending on the organisation. It typically takes 2–3 years to qualify and some courses offer a diploma, while others are certified by the breastfeeding organisation concerned – all are considered comparable.

Breastfeeding counsellors can handle many of the concerns that mums have. Alongside more technical knowledge needed to support breastfeeding, training includes counselling skills to help a mum to explore problems in a safe, non-judgemental space, so that they can find a path forward that works for that particular family.

The vast majority of breastfeeding counsellors are 'employed' in the voluntary sector, so they receive no financial recompense. A small number are employed in peer support schemes or as part of infant feeding teams, but many run support groups, man national helplines, visit the hospital wards or help teach peer supporters in a voluntary capacity.

Lactation consultant

The term lactation consultant loosely refers to anyone working in the field of lactation, either as a volunteer or as a professional, but only the letters IBCLC (International Board Certified Lactation Consultant) after an individual's name show that the person has achieved a recognised standard of independently measured competency in lactation.

IBCLCs have met the criteria to apply for, and passed, the examination set by the International Board of Lactation Consultants Examiners (IBLCE). They are lay health professionals (although some may also be registered health professionals) who specialise in the clinical management of breastfeeding.

Periodic re-certification is mandated by IBLCE, ensuring continuing competence and up-to-date information. IBCLCs may be mothers who have trained as breastfeeding counsellors and served extensively in this role, or they may be midwives or doctors. Both must demonstrate evidence of further study and the required practice hours to apply.

Like most things, however, this system isn't flawless. There has been controversy in recent years over fast access routes to the IBCLC qualification for 'any' health professional, regardless of their level of breastfeeding knowledge (and without having to demonstrate practice hours shadowing a qualified IBCLC), while long-serving breastfeeding counsellors, who are far more knowledgeable, struggle to meet the new strict medical criteria. This means, unfortunately, that IBCLC isn't the guarantee of top-level care that it should be, as some health professionals can take the exam and pass based on their classroom knowledge alone, without any verified practice hours supporting mothers.

Many IBCLCs are employed in the field of clinical lactation and work in hospitals alongside primary healthcare providers, providing training to midwives and peer supporters, or perhaps delivering breastfeeding preparation classes to parents. They may also run support groups or work as I do in private practice, with prices varying across the country.

If we have enough peer supporters and breastfeeding counsellors, we shouldn't need lots of IBCLCs for things to work. It also means that those we do have are being best utilised dealing with more complex cases, rather than doing things others can do perfectly well.

In the UK we have the added complication that we're heavily reliant on the volunteer sector for our breastfeeding support. The National Breastfeeding Helpline is technically funded by the Department of Health, but the funding only covers expenses; those manning it are volunteer breastfeeding counsellors and the maximum they receive in terms of earnings is recompense for any childcare needed during their time answering the telephone. They are not paid healthcare professionals.

In total the helpline took 40,000 calls in 2015. The other breastfeeding support charities took another 10,000 calls between them, and that's not including any of the other work they do (see more below).

Of course, in a funded care system it can be tempting to be short-sighted; to perhaps think that money can be saved by having half the number of IBCLCs and doubling the number of peer supporters. Some areas just have peer supporters, with the only referral options being a GP or health visitor. The thinking seems to be that if everyone works a bit outside of their remit, surely we can fill the gaps? In practice this is not only a false economy, but also not truly supportive or even adequate.

Infant feeding is the cornerstone of health, yet we have voluntary organisations propping up the entire system. If they closed tomorrow, what would happen to breastfeeding rates in the UK? The thousands of calls per year they receive paint a clear picture. Parents not only need appropriately qualified help, but they also need it at the right time to have a chance of succeeding in meeting their breastfeeding goals.

Support needs to be effective and timely

I talk a lot about timely, effective support – but what does it actually mean? Is it a case of telling someone as soon as you have a problem? Partly, yes, but it goes further than this. A skilled breastfeeding supporter should be able to identify a feeding issue within the first few days of life. Often babies aren't massively hungry at birth as they've been nourished continually by the placenta; but by day two appetite can kick in and a baby struggling to feed can become very fussy.

If a problem is identified early, then what? 'Keep at it and things will click...' seems to be the new buzz phrase, in my area at least. It comes into play when a mum has a problem that standard 'positioning and attachment' support doesn't fix and those supporting her are stuck about where to go next. The problem is that this passive stance can have consequences, including damaged nipples, low or static weight gain, a baby never showing signs of being satisfied and a mum who quickly loses confidence.

Unless these mums can find alternative support, I don't see how things will change. Until someone has identified *why* a baby is struggling to feed well, how can we assume it's going to spontaneously resolve? It often doesn't. And a baby can't continue to not gain weight well, any more than a mum can continue feeding 14 hours per day or every half an hour. So the inevitable happens and a formula top-up is suggested, often with a comment along the lines of: 'You've tried this and stuck at it long enough now, you've done really well to get this far, but baby clearly needs more'.

Sometimes the baby gets referred to a paediatrician for low weight gain, despite the fact that nobody has actually checked whether he is taking enough milk. Referral often results in immediate bottle-feeding and cessation of breastfeeding.

Why, when breastfeeding is so important according to every health authority worldwide, are mothers in countries like the UK reporting that they have had insufficient help to succeed? This has to change.

Breastfeeding support
Midwives, health visitors and hospital/local NHS infant
feeding support teams

Voluntary/free-to-user services:
- National Breastfeeding Helpline: 0300 100 0212
- Breastfeeding Network: 0300 100 0210
- La Leche League: 0845 120 2918
- Association of Breastfeeding Mothers: 0300 330 5453
- NCT: 0300 330 0700
- Drugs in Breastmilk Helpline (for parents or
  practitioners to check the safety of a drug for a
  breastfeeding mother): 0844 412 4665.

Private IBCLCs:
- There is no complete list; as all the umbrella
  organisations charge a fee, some practitioners choose
  not to subscribe to some or any of them. The main
  UK database can be found at: www.lcgb.org
- You can also check if someone is an IBCLC simply
  by checking the register at: iblce.org/resources/iblce-
  registry
- My website is www.milkmatters.org.uk

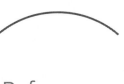

References

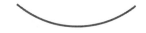

'The Breastcrawl – a scientific overview'. from www.breastcrawl.org

Aarts, C., et al. (1999). 'Breastfeeding patterns in relation to thumb sucking and pacifier use'. *Pediatrics* 104(4): e50.

Abu Raya, B., et al. (2015). 'Optimizing pertussis control among young infants'. *Clin Infect Dis* 60(10): 1587-1588.

Alimoradi, F., et al. (2014). 'An overview of importance of breastfeeding'. *J Compr Ped* 5(2): e14028.

Alm, B., et al. (2002). 'Breast feeding and the sudden infant death syndrome in Scandinavia, 1992–95'. *Arch Dis Child* 86(6): 400-402.

Alvergne, A., et al. (2009). 'Variation in testosterone levels and male reproductive effort: insight from a polygynous human population'. *Horm Behav* 56(5): 491-497.

Anders, T.F. (1979). 'Night-waking in infants during the first year of life'. *Pediatrics* 63(6): 860-864.

Aranda, J.V., et al. (1979). 'Maturation of caffeine elimination in infancy'. *Arch Dis Child* 54(12): 946-949.

Ballard, O. and A. L. Morrow (2013). 'Human milk composition: nutrients and bioactive factors'. *Pediatric Clinics of North America* 60(1): 49-74.

Bartick, M. and A. Reinhold (2010). 'The burden of suboptimal breastfeeding in the United States: a pediatric cost analysis'. *Pediatrics* 125(5): e1048-1056.

Borra, C., et al. (2015). 'New evidence on breastfeeding and postpartum depression: the importance of understanding women's intentions'. *Matern Child Health J* 19(4): 897-907.

Boyd, C.A., et al. (2007). 'Donor breast milk versus infant formula for preterm infants: systematic review and meta-analysis'. *Arch Dis Child Fetal Neonatal Ed* 92(3): F169-175.

Breastfeeding special (2012). 'Breastfeeding and the use of human milk'. *Pediatrics* 129(3): e827-e841.

Bystrova, K., et al. (2003). 'Skin-to-skin contact may reduce negative consequences of 'the stress of being born: a study on temperature in newborn infants, subjected to different ward routines in St. Petersburg'. *Acta Paediatr* 92(3): 320-326.

Cacho, N. and J. Neu (2014). 'Manipulation of the intestinal microbiome in newborn infants'. *Advances in Nutrition: An International Review Journal* 5(1): 114-118.

Carpenter, R.G. and C.W. Shaddick (1965). 'Role of infection, suffocation, and bottle-feeding in cot death; an analysis of some factors in the histories of 110 cases and their controls'. *Br J Prev Soc Med* 19: 1-7.

Carrion, V. and E.A. Egan (1990). 'Prevention of neonatal necrotizing enterocolitis'. *Journal of Pediatric Gastroenterology and Nutrition* 11(3): 317-323.

Chantry, C.J., et al. (2011). 'Excess weight loss in first-born breastfed newborns relates to maternal intrapartum fluid balance'. *Pediatrics* 127(1): e171-179.

Chiesa, C., et al. (2004). 'Diagnosis of neonatal sepsis: a clinical and laboratory challenge'. *Clin Chem* 50(2): 279-287.

Chin, L.Y. and L.H. Amir (2008). 'Survey of patient satisfaction with the Breastfeeding Education and Support Services of The Royal Women's Hospital, Melbourne'. *BMC Health Serv Res* 8: 83.

Cohen Engler, A., et al. (2012). 'Breastfeeding may improve nocturnal sleep and reduce infantile colic: potential role of breast milk melatonin'. *Eur J Pediatr* 171(4): 729-732.

Colaizy, T.T., et al. (2016). 'Impact of optimized breastfeeding on the costs of necrotizing enterocolitis in extremely low birthweight infants'. *J Pediatr*.

Collado, M.C., et al. (2012). 'Microbial ecology and host-microbiota interactions during early life stages'. *Gut Microbes* 3(4): 352-365.

Comina, E., et al. (2006). 'Pacifiers: a microbial reservoir'. *Nurs Health Sci* 8(4): 216-223.

Committee, T.A.o.B.M.P. (2009). ABM Clinical Protocol #3: hospital guidelines for the use of supplementary feedings in the healthy term breastfed neonate. *Breastfeeding Medicine*. 4.

Corvaglia, L., et al. (2013). 'Nonpharmacological management of gastroesophageal reflux in preterm infants'. *Biomed Res Int* 2013: 141967.

Corvaglia, L., et al. (2013). 'Pharmacological therapy of gastroesophageal reflux in preterm infants'. *Gastroenterol Res Pract* 2013: 714564.

Cregan, M.D., et al. (2007). 'Identification of nestin-positive putative mammary stem cells in human breastmilk'. *Cell Tissue Res* 329(1): 129-136.

Cushing, A.H., et al. (1998). 'Breastfeeding reduces risk of respiratory illness in infants'. *Am J Epidemiol* 147(9): 863-870.

da Silveira, L.C., et al. (2009). 'Biofilm formation by Candida species on silicone surfaces and latex pacifier nipples: an in vitro study'. *J Clin Pediatr Dent* 33(3): 235-240.

Daly, S.E. and P.E. Hartmann (1995). 'Infant demand and milk supply. Part 2: The short-term control of milk synthesis in lactating women'. *J Hum Lact* 11(1): 27-37.

Daly, S.E., et al. (1996). 'Frequency and degree of milk removal and the short-term control of human milk synthesis'. *Exp Physiol* 81(5): 861-875.

Das, J.C. (2015). 'Hypernatremic dehydration in newborn infants: a review'. *Ulutas Med J* 1(2): 22-25.

Davis, A.M., et al. (2008). 'Alpha-lactalbumin-rich infant formula fed to healthy term infants in a multicenter study: plasma essential amino acids and gastrointestinal tolerance'. *Eur J Clin Nutr* 62(11): 1294-1301.

Dennis, C.L. and K. McQueen (2009). 'The relationship between infant-feeding outcomes and postpartum depression: a qualitative systematic review'. *Pediatrics* 123(4): e736-751.

Dewey, K.G., et al. (1984). 'Breast milk volume and composition during late lactation (7-20 months)'. *J Pediatr Gastroenterol Nutr* 3(5): 713-720.

Donlan, R.M. (2001). 'Biofilm formation: a clinically relevant microbiological process'. *Clin Infect Dis* 33(8): 1387-1392.

Douglas, P. and P. Hill (2011). 'Managing infants who cry excessively in the first few months of life'. *BMJ* 343: d7772.

Douglas, P.S. (2005). 'Excessive crying and gastro-oesophageal reflux disease in infants: misalignment of biology and culture'. *Med Hypotheses* 64(5): 887-898.

Duncan, J.R., et al. (2010). 'Brainstem serotonergic deficiency in sudden infant death syndrome'. *JAMA* 303(5): 430-437.

Dupont, C., et al. (2010). 'Alpha-lactalbumin-enriched and probiotic-supplemented infant formula in infants with colic: growth and gastrointestinal tolerance'. *Eur J Clin Nutr* 64(7): 765-767.

Edelstein, R.S., et al. (2015). 'Prenatal hormones in first-time expectant parents: Longitudinal changes and within-couple correlations'. *Am J Hum Biol* 27(3): 317-325.

Feldman, R., et al. (2010). 'Natural variations in maternal and paternal care are associated with systematic changes in oxytocin following parent-infant contact'. *Psychoneuroendocrinology* 35(8): 1133-1141.

Ford, R.P., et al. (1993). 'Breastfeeding and the risk of sudden infant death syndrome'. *Int J Epidemiol* 22(5): 885-890.

Foteini, K. and G. Donna (2013). 'Breastmilk composition is dynamic: infant feeds, mother responds'. milkgenomics.org, *The International Milk Genomics Constortium* (IMGC)

Gettler, L.T., et al. (2011). 'Cortisol and testosterone in Filipino young adult men: evidence for co-regulation of both hormones by fatherhood and relationship status'. *Am J Hum Biol* 23(5): 609-620.

Girish, M., et al. (2013). 'Impact and feasibility of breast crawl in a tertiary care hospital'. *J Perinatol* 33(4): 288-291.

Goldberg, W.A., et al. (2013). 'Eye of the beholder? Maternal mental health and the quality of infant sleep'. *Soc Sci Med* 79: 101-108.

Goldman, A.S. (1993). 'The immune system of human milk: antimicrobial, antiinflammatory and immunomodulating properties'. *Pediatr Infect Dis J* 12(8): 664-671.

Goodlin-Jones, B.L., et al. (2001). 'Night waking, sleep-wake organization, and self-soothing in the first year of life'. *J Dev Behav Pediatr* 22(4): 226-233.

Gordon, I., et al. (2010). 'Prolactin, oxytocin, and the development of paternal behavior across the first six months of fatherhood'. *Horm Behav* 58(3): 513-518.

Gray, L., et al. (2000). 'Skin-to-skin contact is analgesic in healthy newborns'. *Pediatrics* 105(1): e14.

Gribble, K.D. (2006). 'Mental health, attachment and breastfeeding: implications for adopted children and their mothers'. *Int Breastfeed J* 1(1): 5.

Gross, A.M. and R.S. Drabman (1990). *Handbook of Clinical Behavioral Pediatrics*, Plenum.

Guaraldi, F. and G. Salvatori (2012). 'Effect of breast and formula feeding on gut microbiota shaping in newborns'. *Front Cell Infect Microbiol* 2: 94.

Hamdan, A. and H. Tamim (2012). 'The relationship between postpartum depression and breastfeeding'. *Int J Psychiatry Med* 43(3): 243-259.

Hanson, L.A. (1998). 'Breastfeeding provides passive and likely long-lasting active immunity'. *Ann Allergy Asthma Immunol* 81(6): 523-533; quiz 533-524, 537.

Hasselbalch, H., et al. (1999). 'Breast-feeding influences thymic size in late infancy'. *Eur J Pediatr* 158(12): 964-967.

Hasselbalch, H., et al. (1996). 'Decreased thymus size in formula-fed infants compared with breastfed infants'. *Acta Paediatr* 85(9): 1029-1032.

Hassiotou, F., et al. (2012). 'Breastmilk is a novel source of stem cells with multilineage differentiation potential'. *Stem Cells* 30(10): 2164-2174.

Hassiotou, F. and D.T. Geddes (2015). 'Immune cell-mediated protection of the mammary gland and the infant during breastfeeding'. *Adv Nutr* 6(3): 267-275.

Hassiotou, F., et al. (2013). 'Cells in human milk: state of the science'. *Journal of Human Lactation*.

Hassiotou, F. and P.E. Hartmann (2014). 'At the dawn of a new discovery: the potential of breast milk stem cells'. *Advances in Nutrition: An International Review Journal* 5(6): 770-778.

Hassiotou, F., et al. (2014). 'Breastmilk stem cell transfer from mother to neonatal organs' (216.4). *The FASEB Journal* 28(1 Supplement).

Hassiotou, F., et al. (2013). 'Maternal and infant infections stimulate a rapid leukocyte response in breastmilk'. *Clin Transl Immunology* 2(4): e3.

Hassiotou, F., et al. (2013). 'Breastmilk cell and fat contents respond similarly to removal of breastmilk by the infant'. *PLoS One* 8(11): e78232.

Hauck, F.R., et al. (2003). 'Sleep environment and the risk of sudden infant death syndrome in an urban population: the Chicago Infant Mortality Study'. *Pediatrics* 111(5 Pt 2): 1207-1214.

Hauck, F.R., et al. (2011). 'Breastfeeding and reduced risk of sudden infant death syndrome: a meta-analysis'. *Pediatrics* 128(1): 103-110.

Hausner, H., et al. (2008). 'Differential transfer of dietary flavour compounds into human breast milk'. *Physiol Behav* 95(1-2): 118-124.

Hausner, H., et al. (2010). 'Breastfeeding facilitates acceptance of a novel dietary flavour compound'. *Clin Nutr* 29(1): 141-148.

Heine, W., et al. (1996). 'alpha-Lactalbumin-enriched low-protein infant formulas: a comparison to breast milk feeding'. *Acta Paediatr* 85(9): 1024-1028.

Heine, W.E. (1999). 'The significance of tryptophan in infant nutrition'. *Adv Exp Med Biol* 467: 705-710.

Hildebrandt, R. and U. Gundert-Remy (1983). 'Lack of pharmacological active saliva levels of caffeine in breast-fed infants'. *Pediatr Pharmacol* (New York) 3(3-4): 237-244.

Hinde, K. and J.B. German (2012). 'Food in an evolutionary context: insights from mother's milk'. *J Sci Food Agric* 92(11): 2219-2223.

Hoffman, H.J., et al. (1988). 'Risk factors for SIDS. Results of the National Institute of Child Health and Human Development SIDS Cooperative Epidemiological Study'. *Ann N Y Acad Sci* 533: 13-30.

Horne, R.S., et al. (2004). 'Comparison of evoked arousability in breast and formula fed infants'. *Arch Dis Child* 89(1): 22-25.

Ip, S., et al. (2007). 'Breastfeeding and maternal and infant health outcomes in developed countries'. *Evid Rep Technol Assess* (Full Rep)(153): 1-186.

J.W, B., et al. (2010) 'Microbial contamination of infant pacifiers: are binkies making baby sick?'

Jackson, K.M. and A.M. Nazar (2006). 'Breastfeeding, the immune response, and long-term health'. *J Am Osteopath Assoc* 106(4): 203-207.

Kantorowska, A., et al. (2016). 'Impact of donor milk availability on breast milk use and necrotizing enterocolitis rates'. *Pediatrics* 137(3): 1-8.

Kendall-Tackett, K. (2007). 'A new paradigm for depression in new mothers: the central role of inflammation and how breastfeeding and anti-inflammatory treatments protect maternal mental health'. *Int Breastfeed J* 2: 6.

Kent, J.C., et al. (2006). 'Volume and frequency of breastfeedings and fat content of breast milk throughout the day'. *Pediatrics* 117(3): e387-395.

Kinney, H.C., et al. (2015). 'Dentate gyrus abnormalities in sudden unexplained death in infants: morphological marker of underlying brain vulnerability'. *Acta Neuropathol* 129(1): 65-80.

Kinney, H.C., et al. (2009). 'The brainstem and serotonin in the sudden infant death syndrome'. *Annu Rev Pathol* 4: 517-550.

Kitzmiller, J. L., et al. (2007). 'Gestational diabetes after delivery: Short-term management and long-term risks'. *Diabetes Care* 30(Supplement 2): S225-S235.

L, S. and P. T (2008). 'Breastfeeding helps prevent two major infant illnesses'. *The Internet Journal of Allied Health Sciences and Practice* 6(3).

Lawrence, R.A. and R.M. Lawrence (2005). *Breastfeeding A Guide For The Medical Profession* Sixth Edition.

Lee, G., et al. (2011). 'Fatherhood, childcare, and testosterone: study authors discuss the details'. scientificamerican.com.

Lehtonen, J., et al. (1998). 'The effect of nursing on the brain activity of the newborn'. *J Pediatr* 132(4): 646-651.

Lien, E.L. (2003). 'Infant formulas with increased concentrations of alpha-lactalbumin'. *Am J Clin Nutr* 77(6): 1555S-1558S.

Lien, E.L., et al. (2004). 'Growth and safety in term infants fed reduced-protein formula with added bovine alpha-lactalbumin'. *J Pediatr Gastroenterol Nutr* 38(2): 170-176.

Lönnerdal, B. (2003). 'Nutritional and physiologic significance of human milk proteins'. *Am J Clin Nutr* 77(6): 1537S-1543S.

Lönnerdal, B. and E.L. Lien (2003). 'Nutritional and physiologic significance of alpha-lactalbumin in infants'. *Nutr Rev* 61(9): 295-305.

Lucas, A. and T.J. Cole (1990). 'Breast milk and neonatal necrotising enterocolitis'. *Lancet* 336(8730): 1519-1523.

Ludington-Hoe, S.M., et al. (2005). 'Skin-to-skin contact (Kangaroo Care) analgesia for preterm infant heel stick'. *AACN Clin Issues* 16(3): 373-387.

Markus, C.R., et al. (2000). 'The bovine protein alpha-lactalbumin increases the plasma ratio of tryptophan to the other large neutral amino acids, and in vulnerable subjects raises brain serotonin activity, reduces cortisol concentration, and improves mood under stress'. *Am J Clin Nutr* 71(6): 1536-1544.

McVea, K.L., et al. (2000). 'The role of breastfeeding in sudden infant death syndrome'. *J Hum Lact* 16(1): 13-20.

Melnik, B.C. (2012). 'Excessive leucine-mtorc1-signalling of cow milk-based infant formula: the missing link to understand early childhood obesity'. *J Obes* 2012: 197653.

Mennella, J.A. (1995). 'Mother's milk: a medium for early flavor experiences'. *J Hum Lact* 11(1): 39-45.

Mennella, J.A. (2006). 'Development of food preferences: lessons learned from longitudinal and experimental studies'. *Food Qual Prefer* 17(7-8): 635-637.

Mennella, J.A. and G.K. Beauchamp (1993). 'The effects of repeated exposure to garlic-flavored milk on the nursling's behavior'. *Pediatr Res* 34(6): 805-808.

Mennella, J.A., et al. (2001). 'Prenatal and postnatal flavor learning by human infants'. *Pediatrics* 107(6): E88.

Mennella, J.A., et al. (1995). 'Garlic ingestion by pregnant women alters the odor of amniotic fluid'. *Chem Senses* 20(2): 207-209.

Mezzacappa, E.S. and E.S. Katlin (2002). 'Breast-feeding is associated with reduced perceived stress and negative mood in mothers'. *Health Psychol* 21(2): 187-193.

Mezzacappa, M.A. and B.G. Ferreira (2016). 'Excessive weight loss in exclusively breastfed full-term newborns in a Baby-Friendly Hospital. *Rev Paul Pediatr.*34(3):281–286.

Mitchell, E.A., et al. (1991). 'Results from the first year of the New Zealand cot death study'. *N Z Med J* 104(906): 71-76.

Mitoulas, L.R., et al. (2002). 'Variation in fat, lactose and protein in human milk over 24h and throughout the first year of lactation'. *Br J Nutr* 88(1): 29-37.

Moimaz, S.A., et al. (2008). 'Association between breast-feeding practices and sucking habits: a cross-sectional study of children in their first year of life'. *J Indian Soc Pedod Prev Dent* 26(3): 102-106.

Mooi, F.R. and S.C. de Greeff (2007). 'The case for maternal vaccination against pertussis'. *Lancet Infect Dis* 7(9): 614-624.

Mosko, S., et al. (1997). 'Maternal proximity and infant CO2 environment during bedsharing and possible implications for SIDS research'. *Am J Phys Anthropol* 103(3): 315-328.

Mulder, E.J., et al. (2010). 'Foetal response to maternal coffee intake: role of habitual versus non-habitual caffeine consumption'. *J Psychopharmacol* 24(11): 1641-1648.

Mulder, P.J., et al. (2010). 'Excessive weight loss in breastfed infants during the postpartum hospitalization'. *J Obstet Gynecol Neonatal Nurs* 39(1): 15-26.

Murray, L., et al. (1996). 'The impact of postnatal depression and associated adversity on early mother-infant interactions and later infant outcome'. *Child Dev* 67(5): 2512-2526.

Neu, J. and W.A. Walker (2011). 'Necrotizing enterocolitis'. *N Eng J Med* 364(3): 255-264.

Ngom, P.T., et al. (2004). 'Improved thymic function in exclusively breastfed infants is associated with higher interleukin 7 concentrations in their mothers' breast milk'. *Am J Clin Nutr* 80(3): 722-728.

Nissen, E., et al. (1996). 'Different patterns of oxytocin, prolactin but not cortisol release during breastfeeding in women delivered by caesarean section or by the vaginal route'. *Early Hum Dev* 45(1-2): 103-118.

Obaro, S.K. (1996). 'Serum, breast milk, and infant antibody after maternal immunisation with pneumococcal vaccine'. *Lancet* 347(8995): 192-193.

Obaro, S.K., et al. (2004). 'Serotype-specific pneumococcal antibodies in breast milk of Gambian women immunized with a pneumococcal polysaccharide vaccine during pregnancy'. *Pediatr Infect Dis J* 23(11): 1023-1029.

O'Brien, E., et al. (2016). 'The portrayal of infant feeding in British women's magazines: a qualitative and quantitative content analysis'. *J Public Health* (Oxf).

Oddy, W.H., et al. (2003). 'Breast feeding and respiratory morbidity in infancy: a birth cohort study'. *Arch Dis Child* 88(3): 224-228.

O'Sullivan, A., et al. (2013). 'Early diet impacts infant rhesus gut microbiome, immunity, and metabolism'. *J Proteome Res* 12(6): 2833-2845.

Palgi, S., et al. (2015). 'Intranasal administration of oxytocin increases compassion toward women. *Soc Cogn Affect Neurosci* 10(3): 311-317.

Palmer, B.D. 'The Importance of Breastfeeding as it Relates to Total Health'. www.brianpalmerdds.com.

Patki, S., et al. (2010). 'Human breast milk is a rich source of multipotent mesenchymal stem cells'. *Hum Cell* 23(2): 35-40.

Preer, G.L., et al. (2012). 'Weight loss in exclusively breastfed infants delivered by cesarean birth'. *J Hum Lact* 28(2): 153-158.

Public Health England (2015). 'New mothers are anxious about breastfeeding in public'. www.gov.uk.

Quigley, M.A., et al. (2007). 'Formula milk versus donor breast milk for feeding preterm or low birth weight infants'. *Cochrane Database Syst Rev*(4): CD002971.

Quigley, M.A., et al. (2007). 'Breastfeeding and hospitalization for diarrheal and respiratory infection in the United Kingdom Millennium Cohort Study'. *Pediatrics* 119(4): e837-842.

Quinello, C., et al. (2010). 'Passive acquisition of protective antibodies reactive with Bordetella pertussis in newborns via placental transfer and breast-feeding'. *Scand J Immunol* 72(1): 66-73.

Rand, S.E. and A. Kolberg (2001). 'Neonatal hypernatremic dehydration secondary to lactation failure'. *J Am Board Fam Pract* 14(2): 155-158.

Redhead, K., et al. (1990). 'Antimicrobial effect of human milk on Bordetella pertussis'. *FEMS Microbiol Lett* 58(3): 269-273.

Renner, J., et al. (2004). 'The relationship between breast size and breast milk volume of nursing primipara'. *Nigerian Quarterly Journal of Hospital Medicine.* 14.

Research, I. (2010). Infant Feeding Survey. U.K.D. Service.

Riskin, A., et al. (2012). 'Changes in immunomodulatory constituents of human milk in response to active infection in the nursing infant'. *Pediatr Res* 71(2): 220-225.

Ruth, L. and L. Robert (2010). 'Breastfeeding: A Guide for the Medical Professional' (Expert Consult - Online and Print).

Ryu, J.E. (1985). 'Effect of maternal caffeine consumption on heart rate and sleep time of breast-fed infants'. *Dev Pharmacol Ther* 8(6): 355-363.

Sadaf, K. (2012). 'Short-term variations in breastmilk composition: associations with feeding patterns and gastric emptying in term infants', University of Western Australia.

Sánchez, C.L., et al. (2009). 'The possible role of human milk nucleotides as sleep inducers. *Nutr Neurosci* 12(1): 2-8.

Sandström, O., et al. (2008). 'Effects of α-lactalbumin–enriched formula containing different concentrations of glycomacropeptide on infant nutrition'. *Am J Clin Nutr* 87(4): 921-928.

Scheele, D., et al. (2013). 'Oxytocin enhances brain reward system responses in men viewing the face of their female partner'. *Proc Natl Acad Sci USA* 110(50): 20308-20313.

Schiff, M., et al. (2014). 'The impact of cosmetic breast implants on breastfeeding: a systematic review and meta-analysis'. *Int Breastfeed J* 9: 17.

Schlaudecker, E.P., et al. (2013). 'IgA and neutralizing antibodies to influenza A virus in human milk: a randomized trial of antenatal influenza immunization'. *PLoS One* 8(8): e70867.

Schurr, P. and E.M. Perkins (2008). 'The relationship between feeding and necrotizing enterocolitis in very low birth weight infants'. *Neonatal Netw* 27(6): 397-407.

Scragg, L. K., et al. (1993). 'Evaluation of the cot death prevention programme in South Auckland'. *N Z Med J* 106(948): 8-10.

Sherman, M.R. (2009). 'Probiotics and Microflora'. *US Pharm.* 2009;34(12):42-44.

Slade, H.B. and S.A. Schwartz (1987). 'Mucosal immunity: the immunology of breast milk'. *J Allergy Clin Immunol* 80(3 Pt 1): 348-358.

SM, A. and K. P (2015). 'Breastfeeding as a tool that empowers infant immunity through maternal vaccination'. *Journal of Vaccines and Vaccination*.

Staub, E. and B. Wilkins (2012). 'A fatal case of hypernatraemic dehydration in a neonate'. *J Paediatr Child Health* 48(9): 859-862.

Steinberg, L.A., et al. (1992). 'Tryptophan intake influences infants' sleep latency'. *J Nutr* 122(9): 1781-1791.

Stuebe, A. (2009). 'The risks of not breastfeeding for mothers and infants'. *Rev Obstet Gynecol* 2(4): 222-231.

Thomas, Jenny M., MPH, IBCLC, FAAP, FABM (2016). 'The normal newborn and why breastmilk is not just food', from www.drjen4kids.com/soap%20box/normal_%20newborn.htm

Trabulsi, J., et al. (2011). 'Effect of an α-lactalbumin-enriched infant formula with lower protein on growth'. *Eur J Clin Nutr* 65(2): 167-174.

Tsopmo, A., et al. (2009). 'Tryptophan released from mother's milk has antioxidant properties'. *Pediatr Res* 66(6): 614-618.

van Amerongen, R.H., et al. (2001). 'Severe hypernatremic dehydration and death in a breast-fed infant'. *Pediatr Emerg Care* 17(3): 175-180.

Van Rie, A., et al. (2005). 'Role of maternal pertussis antibodies in infants'. *Pediatr Infect Dis J* 24(5 Suppl): S62-65.

Vennemann, M.M., et al. (2009). 'Does breastfeeding reduce the risk of sudden infant death syndrome?' *Pediatrics* 123(3): e406-410.

Verd, S., et al. (2015). 'Hospital outcomes of extremely low birth weight infants after introduction of donor milk to supplement mother's milk'. *Breastfeed Med* 10(3): 150-155.

Verduci, E., et al. (2014). 'Epigenetic effects of human breast milk'. *Nutrients* 6(4): 1711-1724.

Vogt, R., et al. (2012). 'Cancer and non-cancer health effects from food contaminant exposures for children and adults in California: a risk assessment'. *Environmental Health* 11(1): 83.

World Health Organization (2003). Global Strategy for Infant and Young Child Feeding.

Williams, A.F., et al. (2007). 'Banking for the future: investing in human milk'. *Arch Dis Child Fetal Neonatal Ed* 92(3): F158-159.

Ystrom, E. (2012). 'Breastfeeding cessation and symptoms of anxiety and depression: a longitudinal cohort study'. *BMC Pregnancy and Childbirth* 12(1): 36.

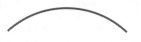

Index